AF527827

Question Bank on Animal Genetics and Breeding

(Course No.: AGB-111, AGB-121 & AGB- 211)

Question Bank on Animal Genetics and Breeding

(Course No.: AGB-111, AGB-121 & AGB- 211)

By :

Dr. Achintya Kumar Das
Principal Scientist

Dr. T.V. Raja
Senior Scientist

Dr. Rajib Deb
Scientist

Dr. Umesh Singh
Principal Scientist

Dr. Sushil Kumar
Principal Scientist

ICAR- Central Institute for Research on Cattle
Grass Farm Road, Post Box No. 17
Meerut Cantt., Meerut - 250001

SSPH

SATISH SERIAL PUBLISHING HOUSE

403, Express Tower, Commercial Complex, Azadpur,
Delhi-110033 (INDIA) Phone : 011-47073040
E-mail : info@satishserial.com, hkjain1975@yahoo.com

Published by :

SATISH SERIAL PUBLISHING HOUSE

403, Express Tower, Commercial Complex, Azadpur,
Delhi-110033 (INDIA) Phone: 011-47073040
E-mail: info@satishserial.com, hkjain1975@yahoo.com

Print Again : 2024

ISBN 978-93-84053-13-0

© 2014. All rights reserved, no part of this publication may be reproduced, stored in a retrieval system or transmitted in any form or by any means, electronic, mechanical, photocopying, recording or otherwise without the prior written permission of the publisher and also the copyright, rights of the printing, publishing, e-book of this edition and subsequent editions will vest with the publisher. All Computer floppies, CD's, e-book and in any other form relating to this book will be exclusive property of the publisher.

This book contains information obtained from authentic and highly regarded sources. Reasonable efforts have been made to publish reliable data and information, but the publisher cannot assume responsibility for the validity of all materials or the consequences of their use. The publisher have attempted to trace and acknowledge the copyright holders of all material reproduced in this publication and apologize to copyright holders if permission and acknowledgements to publish in this form have not been obtained. If any copyright material has not been acknowledged please write and let us know so that we may rectify it.

Composed, Designed & Printed in India

भाकृअनुप
ICAR

केन्द्रीय गोवंष अनुसंधान संस्थान
ICAR-Central Institute for Research on Cattle
(Formerly PD on Cattle)

Dr.B.Prakash
Director

पोस्ट बॉक्स सं. 17, ग्रास फार्म रोड, मेरठ छावनी–250001
PB No. 17, Grass Farm Road, Meerut Cantt.-250001

FOREWORD

I have a great pleasure in forwarding the Question Bank on Animal Genetics and Breeding which is a good attempt of its kind made by the scientists of Animal Genetics & Breeding of this Institute for the use of undergraduate as well as postgraduate students of Animal Genetics and Breeding. This question bank may also be helpful for preparing different competitive exam. like ICAR-JRF, ICAR-SRF, ICAR-NET and ARS.

The mission of the authors will be successful when the students get benefit of such an exhaustive exercise. I am confident that students will find it very useful in understanding and boosting the knowledge of Animal Genetics and Breeding. The effort of the authors in bringing out the book is praiseworthy and I congratulate all of them.

1-10-14

(B. Prakash)

PREFACE

It is the first edition of Question Bank on Animal Genetics and Breeding. It is according to the VCI curriculum after the revised course. This book is designed keeping in mind that the Under Graduate as well as Post Graduate students of Animal Genetics and Breeding can assess this book for regular courses as well as for competitive examination.

Authors extend their sincere thanks to the distinguished authors of various standard text books on Animal Genetics and Breeding and different question banks available in Veterinary sciences.

We extend our gratitude to our Director Dr. B. Prakash for his moral and professional support. We extend our heartiest thanks to all the faculty members of Animal Genetics and Breeding Division, ICAR-CIRC Meerut, for their help and encouragement to bring out this Question Bank.

Achintya Kumar Das
T.V.Raja
Rajib Deb
Umesh Singh
Sushil Kumar

CONTENTS

SECTION-I
AGB-111 : BIOSTATISTICS AND COMPUTER APPLICATION

SECTION-II
AGB-121 : PRINCIPLES OF ANIMAL GENETICS AND POPULATION GENETICS

SECTION-III
AGB-211 : LIVESTOCK AND POULTRY BREEDING

AGB-111 : BIOSTATISTICS AND COMPUTER APPLICATION

Section-I

AGB 111 Biostatistics and Computer Application

1. State True or False

1. When F test is not significant further comparison between means is done by Least Significant Difference test
2. Square of standard error is variance
3. Rejecting the true null hypothesis is called experimental error
4. In a normal distribution, equal number of data lies on either side of mean, median and mode
5. Hard disk is the permanent storage device of a personal computer
6. r_{xy} is equal to r_{yx} but b_{xy} is not equal to b_{yx}
7. Chi-square test is used to compare three means
8. Significant F value indicates existence of difference between all the means in an ANOVA
9. Compact disk is considered as the primary memory of the computer
10. In a positively skewed curve the long tail lies to right side of the curve
11. IN RBD the number of observations in different treatments should always be same
12. Standard deviation is always greater than standard error
13. Regression coefficient and correlation coefficient will have the same signs for same set of data

14. Differences between maximum and minimum values is called coefficient of range
15. As the 'n' increases the SD also increases
16. Number of cows in a farm is an example for continuous variable
17. The reciprocal of standard error is a measure of reliability or precision of the sample
18. Normal distribution is discrete
19. BASIC is a high level language
20. The probability is always a negative fraction
21. Poisson distribution is a probability distribution of economic traits
22. The sum of deviation of observations from mean is always zero
23. Range is the measure of variation which is based on all observations in the series
24. If a constant value 5 is subtracted from each observation of a set, the variance is reduced by 5.
25. Multiplicative law of probability is applicable to independentevents
26. Arithmetic and logical operations are carried out by the monitor
27. Mainframe computers support large number of users simultaneously
28. Windows XP is a hardware
29. Value which is same for all units in the population is termed as a constant
30. Analysis of variance is used to compare three or more groups
31. Square root of variance is called standard error
32. Standard deviation is an absolute measure of dispersion
33. Primary memory of the computer is part of CPU
34. The coefficient of correlation measures not only the magnitude of correlation but also its direction
35. The value of median is determined by each and every observation
36. Smaller the value of variance, greater the uniformity in the population
37. Regression analysis measure the cause-effect relationship between independent and dependent variables

38. In digital computers the data are represented in by a series of 0's and 1's
39. Spread sheets are application software
40. In CRD, all the three principles of experimentations are applied
41. Normal distribution is a Gaussian or symmetrical distribution
42. MS office is an example of computer software
43. When the relationship between more than two variables are studied simultaneously it is called multiple correlation
44. If correlation between two variables is zero, the variables are independent of each other
45. Local control is done to increase the experimental error
46. In ANOVA, 't' test is used to find the significant difference among the sample variances
47. The most accurate method of primary data collection is indirect personal observation
48. Standard deviation can be a negative or positive value
49. The degrees of freedom for chi-square test of independence in a 2x2 contingency table will vary depending upon the nature of data
50. Unlike normal distribution, binomial distribution is the distribution of continuous variable
51. Email is a powerful communication system which can also be used as a search engine
52. In computer software, machine languages are low level languages
53. Calculation of arithmetic mean involves logarithms, making difficulty in calculation
54. In quartile deviation, second quartile is the median
55. Type I error occurs when the null hypothesis is true and our test accepts it
56. SPSS, SAS, MS-Excel are used for carrying out statistical calculations
57. Any computer can be connected with the internet without a modem
58. Pie diagram is the representation of variables by means of bars
59. The unit of expression of correlation coefficient is the unit of dependent variable

60. In normal distribution, equal number of observations lie on either side of mean
61. Standard deviation and standard error can be same for the same set of data
62. Range is the most precise measure of dispersion
63. When one variable decreases 'and if there is a corresponding decrease in the other variable, the correlation coefficient between them will be negative
64. Significant F value in ANOVA, indicates no difference between any two means
65. Regression coefficient can never be negative but correlation coefficient can be negative or positive
66. Rejecting the null hypothesis when it is true is Type I error
67. Mean, median and mode can be same
68. Higher the therapeutic index more will be the safety of a drug
69. bxy is always equal to byx
70. Linux is a computer operating system
71. The null hypothesis is to be rejected when the calculated 't' value is higher than the table 't' value
72. Additive law of probability holds good for mutually exclusive events
73. LD50 is always more than ED50
74. Rectangle in a flowchart indicates processing
75. The standard deviation of data set will not be altered if a constant value is added to all the observations
76. Correlation can be estimated only for the traits which are measured in same units.
77. Kurtosis is the measure of peakedness or convexity of a frequency curve
78. A consistent cricket player will have greater variability in his test scores
79. If the number of replication is increased the experimental error will be reduced.
80. Nonimpact printers generally operate by using a hammer to strike a character against an inked ribbon.

81. Two distributions with same mean and standard deviation should be identical distributions.
82. The range of regression coefficient is -1 to 1.
83. The mainframe computers are used in railway reservation system.
84. In normal distribution, mean ± 2 SD covers 68.27 percentage of data.
85. Student 't' test is the test of choice for comparing three means simultaneously.
86. The data or information sent as an email attachment is also called as hard copy.
87. Secondary data collection is more reliable than primary data collection.
88. ROM requires a steady flow of electricity and so if the power is turned off, the data stored in the ROM will be lost
89. Mode is the middle value and median is the most frequently occurring value
90. The number of items falling in a particular class interval is called as the frequency of that class
91. The computer languages closely resembling the human language are known as high level language
92. In a table, footnote is always given at the top following the heading
93. In percentage bar diagram the height of the bars are always equal
94. Estimate is the value of a population parameter obtained from the sample
95. Binomial distribution is the distribution of continuous variable
96. Ogive is the graphical representation of the cumulative frequency distribution
97. Hybrid computer is suitable combination of both digital and analog computers
98. Product of two regression coefficients is equal to the square of the correlation coefficient
99. Laser printer is an impact printer
100. Geometric mean of a data series will be zero if one or more values is zero
101. The probability of all possible outcomes of a random experiment is always equal to one

102. To study the animal or human population, sampling method gives the accurate result than the census method
103. Hard copy is a printed copy of information from a computer.
104. Range is not affected by extreme values.
105. A bit consists of 8 bytes.
106. Secondary data can be accepted without further scrutiny.
107. The geometric mean cannot be calculated if one or more values in a series is negative
108. The scanner is an output device.
109. Animal census is conducted once in 10 years.
110. In flow chart, the process of following two or more alternative paths of computation is known as branching
111. Internet is the world's largest network of computers
112. Data base query languages and report generators are examples of nonprocedural languages
113. Cubes, cylinders and spheres are examples of two dimensional diagrams
114. Correlation and regression coefficients are the same when variances of X and Y are different.
115. Regression coefficient is an absolute measure.
116. The ratio of LD50 to ED50 is called as therapeutic index.
117. Rejecting the true null hypothesis is called experimental error.
118. ED50 of a drug should be as high as possible to consider it to be effective.
119. In test of significance, if calculated value is less than the theoretical value, we accept null hypothesis.
120. Given the same data, outcomes can be significant at the 0.01 level but not at the 0.05 level.
121. Local Area Network (LAN) is a computer network that spans a relatively small area
122. The storage capacity of 3 1/2" floppy is 1.44 MB
123. If A and B are two independent events, then P(AB) = P(A) P(B)
124. Mode is not suitable for further algebraic operations

125. If the number of observations increases the standard error also increases
126. When type I error occurs, type II error cannot occur simultaneously
127. Harmonic mean is always greater than geometric mean
128. Geometric mean is suitable for testing averages of ratios and percentages
129. In open end classes the lower limit of the last class and upper limit of the first class are not defined
130. The statistical procedures which deals with collection, classification and tabulation of data is known as inferential statistics
131. Standard deviation is the negative root of variance
132. Second quartile is known as median
133. Key board is an output device
134. The most ideal measure of central tendency is mode
135. Moment is a term which refers to the measure of a force with respect to its tendency to provide rotation
136. Probability lies between 0 to 1
137. The third moment about the mean measures Kurtosis
138. The set of all possible outcomes of a random experiment is known as sample space
139. Baye's theorem helps to measure the conditional probability
140. The result of parametric tests is more reliable and powerful than the non-parametric tests
141. In case of regression both the variables are independent of each other.
142. Formula for chi–square test is $\frac{\sum(E-O)^2}{E}$
143. Chi-square was given by R.A.Fisher.
144. Regression coefficient is independent of scale and origin.
145. Relationship between three types of means is GM $\geq$ AM $\geq$ HM.
146. Standard deviation is a measure of reliability of an estimate.
147. Significance of coefficient of relation is tested by chi-square test.
148. Coefficient of variation will be 5% in case mean & variance are 40 gm & $4g^2$ respectively.

149. If potency of drug is low, its therapeutic dose will be very high.

150. Therapeutic index of a drug is ratio of ED_{50}/LD_{50}.

151. Mode = 3 Median – 2 Mean.

152. When data amount is same, the Completely Randomised Design will have higher error degrees of freedom then the Randomised Block Design.

153. In experimental design the principle of local control is applied to minimize the experimental error.

154. A null hypothesis is rejected at 1% significance level means, it will be definitely rejected at 5% level.

155. Square of regression coefficient is called as coefficient of determination.

156. The axiomatic theory of probability was given by Simon de Laplace.

157. The probability of getting at least one head in two successive toss of coin is equal to 0.5.

158. In exceptional cases the value of probability of an event can be 1.01.

159. The number of ways "r" objects can be selected from "n" objects is P (n,r).

160. Analog computer uses binary numbers for operations.

161. In case of regression both the variables are independent of each other.

162. Square of regression coefficient is called as coefficient of determination.

163. Chi-square was given by R.A. Fisher.

164. Regression coefficient is independent of scale and origin.

165. Relationship between three types of means is GM ≥ AM ≥ HM.

166. Standard deviation is a measure of reliability of an estimate.

167. Significance of coefficient of relation is tested by chi-square test.

168. Coefficient of variation will be 5% in case mean & variance are 40 & 42 gms, respectively.

169. If potency of drug is low, its therapeutic dose will be very high.

170. A null hypothesis is rejected at 1% significance level means, it will be definitely rejected at 5% level.

KEY

1.	False	2.	False
3.	False	4.	True
5.	True	6.	True
7.	False	8.	False
9.	False	10.	True
11.	True	12.	True
13.	True	14.	False
15.	False	16.	False
17.	True	18.	False
19.	True	20.	False
21.	False	22.	True
23.	False	24.	False
25.	True	26.	False
27.	True	28.	False
29.	True	30.	True
31.	False	32.	True
33.	True	34.	True
35.	False	36.	True
37.	True	38.	True
39.	True	40.	False
41.	True	42.	True
43.	True	44.	True
45.	False	46.	False
47.	False	48.	False
49.	False	50.	False
51.	False	52.	True
53.	False	54.	True
55.	False	56.	True
57.	False	58.	False
59.	False	60.	True
61.	False	62.	False
63.	False	64.	False

65.	False	66.	True
67.	True	68.	True
69.	False	70.	True
71.	True	72.	True
73.	True	74.	True
75.	True	76.	False
77.	True	78.	False
79.	False	80.	False
81.	False	82.	False
83.	True	84.	False
85.	False	86.	False
87.	False	88.	False
89.	False	90.	True
91.	True	92.	False
93.	True	94.	True
95.	False	96.	True
97.	True	98.	True
99.	False	100.	True
101.	True	102.	False
103.	True	104.	False
105.	False	106.	False
107.	True	108.	False
109.	False	110.	True
111.	True	112.	True
113.	False	114.	False
115.	True	116.	True
117.	True	118.	False
119.	True	120.	False
121.	True	122.	True
123.	True	124.	True
125.	True	126.	True
127.	False	128.	True
129.	False	130.	False

131.	False	132.	True
133.	False	134.	False
135.	True	136.	True
137.	False	138.	True
139.	True	140.	True
141.	False	142.	False
143.	False	144.	False
145.	False	146.	False
147.	False	148.	True
149.	True	150.	False
151.	True	152.	True
153.	True	154.	False
155.	False	156.	False
157.	False	158.	False
159.	False	160.	False
161.	False	162.	False
163.	False	164.	False
165.	False	166.	False
167.	False	168.	False
169.	True	170.	False

2. Fill up the Blanks with Suitable Answer

1. The product of regression coefficients is the square of ______________
2. In a calving, the probability of getting a male calf is ______________
3. In a sampling distribution, if the acceptance region is 95%, the critical region will be ______________
4. The act of making and recording a measurement is called ______________
5. Sample A has 10 observations and sample B has 15 observations. The d.f. for finding the table 't' value is ______________
6. In a 3 x 3 contingency table for chi-square test, the d.f. is ______________
7. The law of probability for mutually exclusive event is ______________ and that for independent events is ______________

8. The standard deviation of sample mean is called ________________
9. Less than cumulative frequency relates to the ________________ limit of the class interval
10. In an oil refinery where flows of temperature and measurements are important ________________ type of computers are used.
11. Presentation of data in the form of maps is known as ________________
12. ________________ is the representative of the population
13. The class having maximum frequency is known as ________________ class
14. The speed of super computers are measured in terms of ________________ while the speed of traditional computers are measured as ________________
15. The average of upper and lower limit of a class is known as ________________
16. Published reports are ________________ source of data
17. Paired 't' test is applicable only when the observations are ________________
18. In normal distribution, mean ± SD includes ________________ per cent of observations
19. If one of the regression is greater than one the other will be ________________
20. If all the events have equal chance of occurrence, then these events are said to be ________________
21. Mean, median and mode coincides in case of ________________ distribution
22. Root mean squared deviation is called ________________
23. The difference between maximum and minimum value is known as ________________
24. The probability of impossible event is ________________
25. Ordered arrangement of objects is known as ________________ while unordered arrangement is called as ________________
26. The statistical measure which describes the sample is known as ________________

27. In an asymmetric distribution longer tail towards left is known as ______________________

28. Compact disk is a ________________ storage device

29. ____________________ is the measure of peakedness of the population

30. The primary objective of blocking in an experimental design is to reduce ________________

31. In bioassay, the shape of quantal dose response curve will be __________________

32. The statistical tests which make certain assumptions about the parameters of the population from which the sample is taken are known as ________________

33. The harmonic mean is the _______________ of the arithmetic mean of the reciprocal of the observations.

34. In a 3 x 2 contingency table the d.f. is ________________a

35. ______________ measures the shape of the curve

36. ______________ is the temporary memory of the computer

37. To obtain F value in an ANOVA table, the MSS of the treatment should be divided by the ____________________

38. A bar diagram in which all the bars will be of same height always, is known as ___________________

39. One maga byte is equal to ____________ kilobytes

40. Ratio of standard deviation and mean expressed in percentage is __________________

41. Comparison of means of two large samples is done by _____________

42. The F value is considered as significant if the calculated value is ________________ than table value

43. Any numerical property, characteristic or fact that is descriptive of a population is called as ___________________

44. Visual display unit is an example for ___________________ device

45. The systematic arrangement of data in rows and columns is known as________________

46. Black box in airplane is an example for ______________________ computer

47. The value which remains unchanged throughout the program is called ________________

48. ________________________ is the geometric mean of two regression coefficients

49. The statistical design that allows unequal number of replications of treatment is ____________________.

50. If three cows in a dairy farm have calved on the same day, the probability of all the three calves being female is ___________________.

51. _____________ is the form of experiment for the estimation of potency of a substance.

52. The measure to study the coefficient of correlation between two qualitative characters is ___________________

53. The program that translate the whole program of source code at once into machine language is called __________________

54. Pictorial representation of the logical flow of data or algorithm of a program is known as _______________________

55. The first generation computers were powered by _________________

56. High level languages viz., FORTRAN, COBOL, BASIC etc. were developed and came into operation during __________________ generation of computer

57. If the occurrence of one event prevents the occurrence of another event, they are said to be ________________ events.

58. The DOS command used to rename a file is _____________

59. The mean, median and mode of data series of -3,-3,3,0,0,0,3 are ___________, _____________ and ____________.

60. __________________ variable is the one which cannot be measured and expressed in magnitude

61. The only programming language that computer can understand is ________________

62. If the body weight of five calves were 25 kg each, then the standard deviation will be _______________

63. The curve of normal distribution is _____________ shaped

64. Bar code reader is an _____________ device

65. The single value which is used to estimate the population parameter is known as ____________________ while ________________ estimate gives the limit with in which the population parameter lies

66. In a CRD with 6 treatments each replicated 5 times, the degrees of freedom for error is ______________

67. The ratio of LD50 to ED50 is called as __________________

68. __________________ or ________________ keys of the keyboard can be used to get the uppercase letters in a computer

69. The most useful and popularly used measure of dispersion is ____________________.

70. The sum of deviations of all the observations from the mean is equal to ____________________.

71. In open end classes ______________ limit of the first class and _______________ limit of the last class are not specified.

72. The unit of CPU, called as brain of the computer is _______________.

73. In tabulation, column heading is known as __________________ while the row heading is known as _______________

74. The square of correlation coefficient is known as ___________________ which is used to study the accuracy of statistical analysis

75. The touch pad is an ____________________ device.

76. The distribution of rare occurrences is called ____________________

77. ______________ presentation is a widely used tool in MS-Office which has replaced overhead and slide projectors.

78. _______________ translates a computer program into machine language one line at a time, executing each line of the program after it is translated

79. Regression analysis can be used for prediction of _______________ variable from the known _______________ variable

80. Performing a random experiment is known as _________________ and its outcome is called __________________

81. The analysis of variance technique was given by _______________

82. If a curve is more flatter than the normal distribution curve, it is called __________________

83. Under ____________ method, data are collected from each and every unit of the universe
84. Probability value ranges between ____________ and ___________
85. If the amount of change in one variable tends to bear a constant ratio to the amount of change in the other variable, the correlation is said to be ______________
86. Rejection of a true null hypothesis leads to _______________ error.
87. The shape of graded response curve is _______________
88. The diagrammatic method of studying correlation is _______________
89. Animal or group of animals subjected to treatment is called _______________
90. If the occurrence of one event in no way affects the occurrence of another event, then these events are _______________
91. Large sample test is done when the sample size is _______________
92. The diamond symbol in flow chart is used to denote _______________
93. If the correlation coefficient is zero, the value of regression coefficient is _______________
94. Body weight in goats follows _______________ distribution.
95. By joining the mid points on the upper sides of the adjacent rectangles of the histogram with a straight line , we obtain _________________
96. Two commonly used computer operating systems are _____________ and __________________.
97. All the calculations and comparisons are made in the _____________ unit of the CPU
98. ______________ test is conducted to find the goodness of fit and test of independence
99. If two variables X and Y are independent, the correlation coefficient will be __________________.
100. ______________________ is a specific form of bioassay which involves the matching of the material of unknown potency with an international or national standard with an objective of providing a preparation for use in therapeutics
101. ________ and _______ are the visual form of representing the data

102. The probability of getting a king or queen if one card is drawn from a standard pack of 52 is ____________

103. Presentation of data in the form of pictures is known as __________________ (Pictogram)

104. Acceptance of a false null hypothesis leads to ______________ error.

105. __________________ is used as a measure of variation to compare two sets of data expressed in different units of measurements.

106. __________________ variable is the one which cannot be measured and expressed in magnitude

107. The purposive, quota sampling etc. are ______________ sampling methods

108. Among 100 animals with average Hb of 10 gm%, the standard deviation was 1, the standard error is ___________.

109. In an experiment, the process of repeated application of the treatments under investigation to the experimental units is known as __________________

110. In a computer program, executing a statement or a group of statements for a number of times is called ______________

111. In LAN computers are connected to each other by means of __________________

112. The test of significance used in an RBD design is ________________

113. The Classification of data according to the place of occurrence is known as ______________________

114. Milk production is an example for _____________ variable

115. For any distribution the sum of deviations taken from the arithmetic mean will be _________________

116. _________________ originated in 1969, through a project called ARPANET (Advanced Research Project Agency Network) started by the Department of Defence DOD) of USA.

117. 95 % of the area under a normal curve lies between the limits ______________ region

118. For testing equality of two variances we use _____________ test

119. In design of experiment, random allotment of treatment to the experimental units is known as ____________________

120. Google, yahoo etc. are ________________ commonly used as an interactive tool to help people locate information available in the internet

121. Spearman's rank correlation test is an example for ________________ test

122. The third generation computer languages are known as __________ while the fourth generation languages are ________________

123. Coefficient of correlation lies between _____________ and _____________

124. The two types of primary storage or memory units are ______________ and _______________

125. ________________ is called heart and nerve centre of the computer

126. Local control is also known as ________________

127. In CRD the experimental material should be _______________

128. ______________ is the arithmetic mean of the squares of sum of deviations from the mean value of the data

129. The Poisson distribution takes values from _____________ to __________

130. ______________ is known as father of computer

131. CPU consists of ____________ , ____________ and ____________ units

132. Key board is an __________ unit

133. Occurrence of two or more simple events simultaneously is called as __________________

134. ______________ is equal to square of the standard deviation

135. If regression of X on Y is negative, then the regression of Y on X should be ___________

136. The test of significance applied for related variables is ____________

137. A byte is made up of _____

138. The graphic representation of frequencies or relative frequencies of a continuous quantitative data in the form of bars is ______________

139. The formula for estimating the standard error is _____________

140. In a negatively skewed distribution, the relationship between mean, median and mode is ______________________

141. In the denotation of a websites 'www' stands for ________________.

142. Write the name of the text book _________________________ with author(s) you have referred for the AGB-111 ____________________

143. Root mean square deviations is known as________________ of a population sample.

144. Sum of squares of observations and square of sum of observations is represented as____________ and ____________ respectively.

145. Statistics obtained from a random sample of a population is an_________________.

146. F- Test is also known as________________ test and was devised by___________.

147. Name three computer languages _________, ________________ and ________________ .

148. Mean, mode, and median lies at the same point in_______________ Distribution

149. ____________ is the technique of partitioning of variation into different components

150. The co-efficient of correlation is estimated from a sample of _____________ population

151. ____________ Test is used for testing the significance of correlation co-efficient

152. In hypothesis testing we commit type I error by ____________ when it is true.

153. Optic Pen is an_____________ device.

154. The Mean of Normal Distribution is 50, its mode will be _________

155. Concept of coefficient of correlation was given by ______________

KEY

1. Correlation coefficient
2. ½
3. 5%
4. Observation
5. 23
6. 4

7. Additive, multiplicative
8. Standard error
9. Upper
10. Analog
11. Cartogram
12. Sample
13. Modal
14. Million operations per second, Million instructions per second
15. Mid value
16. Secondary
17. Dependent
18. 68.27
19. Lesser than one
20. Equally likely
21. Normal/ symmetrical
22. Standard deviation
23. Range
24. Zero
25. Permutation, Combination
26. Statistic
27. Negative skewness
28. Secondary
29. Kurtosis
30. Experimental error
31. Normal Bell shaped
32. Parametric tests
33. Reciprocal
34. Two
35. Skewness
36. RAM
37. Error MSS
38. Percentage bar diargam
39. 1024KB
40. Coefficient of variation
41. Z-test
42. Higher/ more
43. Parameter
44. Output
45. Tabulation
46. Special purpose digital
47. constant
48. Correlation coefficient
49. Completely Randomized Design (CRD)
50. 1/851.
Bioassay
52. Spearman's rank correlation
53. Compiler
54. Flow chart
55. Vacuum tubes
56. Second
57. Mutually exclusive
58. REN
59. 0,0,0
60. Qualitative
61. Machine language/ low level language
62. Zero
63. Bell

64. Input
65. Point estimate, interval
66. 24
67. Therapeutic index
68. Shift, caps lock
69. Standard deviation
70. Zero
71. Lower, upper
72. Control Unit
73. Caption, Stub
74. Coefficient of determination (R^2)
75. Input
76. Poisson distribution
77. Power point
78. Interpreter
79. Dependent, independent
80. Trial, event
81. Fisher
82. Platykurtic
83. Census
84. 0 to 1
85. Linear
86. Type I error.
87. Sygmoid or S shaped
88. Scatter diagram
89. Experimental unit
90. Independent events
91. More than 30
92. Decision
93. Zero
94. Continuous normal distribution
95. Frequency polygon
96. MS DOS, Linux and Windows
97. Arithmetic and Logic Unit
98. Chi-square
99. Zero
100. Biological standardization
101. Diagrams and graphs
102. 8/52 or 2/13
103. Pictogram
104. Type II
105. Coefficient of variation
106. Qualitative
107. Non random
108. 0.1
109. Replication
110. Looping
111. Cables
112. F test
113. Geographical or spatial classification
114. Continuous
115. Zero
116. Internet
117. Acceptance
118. F test
119. Randomization
120. Search engines
121. Non-parametric
122. Procedural, Problem oriented
123. -1 to +1

124. RAM and ROM
125. Central Processing Unit
126. Blocking
127. Homogenous
128. Variance
129. 0 to μ
130. Charles Babbage
131. ALU, CU and Primary storage unit /Memory unit
132. Input
133. Mixed or compound or joint events
134. Variance
135. Negative
136. Paired 't' test
137. 8 bits
138. Histogram
139. SD/Ön
140. Mean<Median<Mode
141. World wide web
142.
143. Standard deviation
144. ΣX^2 and $(\Sigma X)^2$
145. Estimate
146. Variance, Fisher
147. Coral C++, Fortran
148. Normal
149. ANOVA
150. Two
151. 't'
152. Rejecting null hypothesis
153. Input
154. 50
155. Karl Person

3. Choose the Most Appropriate Answer

1. The variable which can take any numerical value within certain range is

    a) Continuous variable b) Constant
    c) Parameter d) Discrete variable

2. When two variables move in the same direction, the relationship between them is called

    a) Negative correlation b) Zero correlation
    c) Positive correlation d) Multiple correlation

3. In a simple regression equation of Y = a+ b X, a represents

    a) Regression coefficient b) Slope of regression line
    c) Correlation coefficient d) Intercept

4. The measure of central tendency which divides the data into two equal parts is

   a) Mode b) Median
   c) Peak value d) Arithmetic mean

5. In computer terminology a set of instructions is called

   a) Hardware b) Program
   c) Command d) Language

6. Grouping of homogenous experimental units into blocks is known as

   a) Replication b) Experimental error
   c) Local control d) Randomization

7. One of the following is not a Boolean operator

   a) AND b) NOT
   c) TO d) OR

8. The second moment about the mean measures

   a) Skewness b) Arithmetic Mean
   c) Variance d) Kurtosis

9. Find out the odd one in the list given below

   a) Monitor b) Touch pad
   c) Mouse d) Key board

10. Components of a sample space are known as

    a) Sample points b) Null sets
    c) Simple events d) Compound events

11. In flow charts parallelogram symbol is used to indicate

    a) Input b) Decision
    c) Connector d) Process

12. One Giga byte is equal to

    a) 1024 byte b) 1024 KB
    c) 1024 MB d) 2^{40} Byte

13. An example for a continuous variable is

a) Sex b) Blood group
c) Hair color d) Height

14. The largest, fastest and most expensive computers used in space, petroleum engineering, defense research etc. are

a) Mainframe computers b) Super computers
c) Microcomputers d) Minicomputers

15. The ordered arrangements of the objects is called

a) Ordering b) Combination
c) Arrangement d) Permutation

16. The distribution in which the mean, median and mode coincide is

a) Positively skewed b) Negatively skewed
c) Symmetrical d) Asymmetrical

17. A group of 8 bits is called

a) Byte b) Boot
c) Mega Byte d) None of the above

18. Classification of data based on the time of occurrence is called

a) Quantitative classification b) Geographical classification
c) Spatial classification d) Chronological classification

19. The CPU of the personal computer consists of

a) Memory Unit b) Arithmetic and logic unit
c) Control Unit d) All the above

20. The value laying half way between the lower and upper limit of the class is

a) Class limit b) Mid value
c) Class interval d) Class width

21. The test used for finding the significance of difference between the means of two dependent samples is

a) Z - test b) t-test
c) F-test d) Paired t-test

22. The measure of a force with respect to its tendency to provide rotation is termed as

a) Energy
b) Moments
c) Skewness
d) Kurtosis

23. The speed of a computer processor is measured in

a) Mhz
b) MB
c) KB
d) Frequency

24. The nonparametric test is

a) Z-test
b) Chi-square test
c) F-test
d) t-test

25. Performing a random experiment is called as

a) Event
b) Outcome
c) Trial
d) Probability

26. Which of the following is not a diagrammatic representation of data

a) Histogram
b) Pictogram
c) Bar diagram
d) Cartogram

27. Output of a computer in the form of a printout is otherwise called

a) Soft copy
b) Hard ware
c) Hard copy
d) Hard disk

28. If the standard deviation is 0.5, then the variance is

a) 0.25
b) 0.025
c) 0.70
d) 0.20

29. Which of the following is not a relational operator

a) =
b) ^
c) <=
d) >

30. Computerized DBMS for capturing, storing, analyzing and displaying data related to the locations is known as

a) Browsing
b) National Informaticcentre
c) Geographical information system
d) None of the above

31. Find out the odd one in the given list

a) Quartile deviation
b) Range
c) Median
d) Mean deviation

32. The arithmetic mean of four numbers is 13. Three of the numbers are 5, 13 and 10. The fourth number is

a) 13
b) 20
c) 24
d) 12

33. The normal bell shaped distribution curve is

a) Platykurtic
b) Normokurtic
c) Mesokurtic
d) Leptokurtic

34. For a set of 20 observations, if the mean is 6 and standard deviation is 3 then the coefficient of variation is

a) 40 %
b) 16%
c) 50 %
d) 32 %

35. As per the hierarchy of arithmetic operations in computer programming, which of the following sequences is correct

a) * / + -
b) - + / *
c) / * - +
d) * + / _

36. In order to test whether the data on progeny of a trihybrid cross is following the expected ratio or not, we use

a) t-test
b) F-test
c) Z-test
d) Chi-square test

37. The precision of an experiment can be raised by

a) Increasing the number of treatments
b) Increasing number of replications
c) Decreasing number of treatments
d) Decreasing number of replications

38. The generation of computers in which microprocessor is used

a) First
b) Third
c) Fourth
d) Second

39. The second quartile Q_2 is the

a) Median
b) Mode
c) Deviation
d) Mean

40. The graphical representation of a cumulative frequency distribution is

a) Histogram
b) Scatter plot
c) Ogive
d) Pie diagram

41. In a symmetrical distribution the relationship between arithmetic mean, median and mode is

a) AM = Median = Mode
b) AM < Median < Mode
c) AM > Median > Mode
d) AM <Mode > Median

42. The third moment about the mean measures

a) Skewness
b) Mean
c) Variance
d) Kurtosis

43. In normal distribution the observations covered by mean ± 2 S.D is

a) 68.27%
b) 99.73 %
c) 50.00%
d) 95.45%

44. The type of variable which ends with the % sign is

a) Single precision variable
b) Double precision variable
c) Integer variable
d) String variable

45. The program that translate the whole program of source code at once into machine language is called

a) Interpreter
b) Compiler
c) Processor
d) Transistor

46. The speed of super computers is measured as

a) Million instructions per second
b) Mhz
c) Million operations per second
d) None of the above

47. The various physical components of a computer consisting of electronic and mechanical devices which can be seen and touch are known as

a) Softwares b) Hardwares
c) Firmwares d) None of the above

48. Compiler, assembler, interpreter etc. are examples of

a) System software b) Application software
c) Hardware d) None of the above

49. Laser printer is an example for

a) Impact printer b) Line printer
c) Nonimpact printer d) None of the above

50. Mean is a measure of

a) Location (central value) b) Dispersion
c) Correlation d) None of the above

51. The type of computers used in the banks are

a) Mainframe computers b) Super computers
c) Mini computers d) None of the above

52. If expected and observed frequencies of classes are same, the chi-square value will be

a) μ b) + 1
c) - 1 d) 0

53. The first generation computers were powered by

a) Vacuum tubes b) Steam engines
c) Transistors d) None of the above

54. Dot matrix printer is an example for

a) Line printer b) Impact printer
c) Both a and b d) None of the above

55. The degrees of freedom for statistic-t for paired t-test based on n pairs of observations is

a) 2 (n-1) b) n-1
c) 2n-1 d) None of the above

56. In computer programming double precision variables are denoted by

a) # sign
b) !sign
c) @ sign
d) % sign

57. The fifth generation computer languages are known as

a) Machine languages
b) Procedural languages
c) Problem oriented languages
d) Natural languages

58. In computer programming the sign equal to (=) is a

a) Boolean operator
b) Relational operator
c) Both a and b
d) None of the above

59. The visual display unit, CD, DVD, pen drive etc. are

a) Secondary storage devices
b) Softcopy devices
c) Both a and b
d) None of the above

60. Paired t-test is applicable when observations in two samples are

a) Equal in number
b) Correlated
c) Paired
d) All the above

61. If occurrence of an event prevent occurrence of other they are said to be

a) Equally likely
b) Independent
c) Mutually exclusive
d) Exhaustive

62. The variable whose value is influenced by other variable is called ..... Variable

a) Dependent
b) Exhaustive
c) Random
d) None of the above

63. The application of statistical methods in biological science is called as

a) Biostatistics
b) Inferential statistics
c) Descriptive statistics
d) None of the above

64. Which of the following can be used when positive and negative values are present in the data

a) Harmonic mean
b) Geometric mean
c) Both of the above
d) None of the above

65. Which of the following central tendency is not based on all observations

a) Mean b) Mode
c) Range d) Harmonic mean

66. Statistical method used to compare two or more samples simultaneously is

a) t-test b) ANOVA
c) Regression d) Correlation

67. In statistics, the aggregate from which the sample is to be taken is known as

a) Census b) Sampling
c) Data d) Universe

68. Which of the following is an assumption in data used for 't' test

a) Random b) Continuous
c) Normal d) All the above

69. If number of trials is large and probability of occurrence of an event is very small, the distribution is

a) Normal b) Binomial
c) Poisson d) None of the three

70. If a coin is tossed twice, the result of second throw would not affect the result of first throw and this type of events are

a) Mutually exclusive b) Compound
c) Equally likely d) Independent events

71. Who is the father of biometry, biostatistics and Eugenics

a) Francis Galton b) Gregor Mendel
c) Charles Darwin d) Robert Bakewell

72. The statistical measure computed from a sample

a) Parameter b) Variable
c) Statistic d) Constant

73. Among the following which is not an online input device

a) Mouse b) Key board
c) Pen drive d) Touch pad

74. The relationship between milk yield and fat yield in cattle is an example for

a) Positive correlation
b) Spurious correlation
c) Zero correlation
d) Negative correlation

75. The test where the deviation from a hypothetical ratio is reduced to a single value

a) F test
b) t Test
c) Z test
d) Chi-square test

76. A premier S & T organization of Government of India in the field of Information services and Information Technology application

a) CSIR
b) Infosys
c) Techno park
d) NIC

77. The part of the central processing unit of a computer that performs fundamental mathematical and logical operations is

a) ROM
b) Key board
c) ALU
d) RAM

78. A computer language that is made up of 'zeros' and 'ones' is

a) Machine language
b) BASIC
c) Problem Oriented language
d) C++

79. Accuracy of a computer is very high. Still errors can occur. If a wrong input is given, the out pout put will be wrong. Which of the following term expresses this feature of the computers?

a) Recycle Bin
b) GOGO
c) GIGO
d) Delete

80. The volatile memory of the computer is

a) ROM
b) RAM
c) CD-ROM
d) CPU

81. The programming language one combines the features of

a) COBOL and FORTRAN
b) PASCAL and BASIC
c) BASIC and COBOL
d) BASIC and FORTRAN

82. The statistical test of significance using variance of the data is

a) F test
b) Chi-square test
c) t test
d) z test

83. In an experiment with Completely Randomised Design, number of treatments was 5 and total experimental units used were 30. What is the error degrees of freedom?

a) 3
b) 25
c) 29
d) None of above

84. The most suitable measure of central tendency when small values need be given higher weightage is

a) Arithmetic Mean
b) Geometric mean
c) Harmonic mean
d) Weighted Arithmetic Mean

85. In normal distribution

a) Mean = Median
b) Mean >Median
c) Mean < Median
d) Any of the above

86. When all the observations are same the standard deviation is

a) Zero
b) One
c) Infinity
d) None of the above

87. Coefficient of variation ranges between

a) -1 and +1
b) Zero and 100
c) 1 and 2
d) - 8 and + 8

88. Sampling in which data is obtained by selecting every n^{th} object is

a) Systematic sampling
b) Cluster sampling
c) Stratified sampling
d) None of the above

89. Permanent storage device in a computer is

a) Hard disk
b) Clip board
c) Mother board
d) None of the above

90. The relative measure of dispersion is

a) Range
b) Standard deviation
c) Coefficient of variation
d) Mean deviation

91. The measure of dispersion free from unit and scale of measurement is
    a) Coefficient of variation b) Mean deviation
    c) Arithmetic mean d) Variance

92. Diagrammatic representation of data includes
    a) Bar and area diagram b) Pie diagram
    c) Divided bar diagram d) All the above

93. The analysis of variance technique was given by
    a) Karl Pearson b) Galton
    c) Fisher d) Wright

94. Method used for formation of frequency distribution
    a) Census method b) Random table
    c) Array method d) None of the above

95. Cumulative frequency curve
    a) Ogive b) Histogram
    c) Frequency polygon d) Frequency curve

96. Single value to estimate the parameter
    a) Range b) Estimator
    c) Interval estimate d) Point estimate

97. Non-parametric test
    a) Large sample test b) t-test
    c) Sign test d) F-test

98. In flow chart the rounded rectangle denotes
    a) Start or stop b) Decision
    c) Process d) All the above

99. Which of the following is a squared unit measure of dispersion?
    a) Standard deviation b) Coefficient of variation
    c) Variance d) Standard error

c) Variance   d) Standard error

100. In case of negatively skewed distribution, the relation between mean, median and mode is

a) Mean=median=mode   b) Mean<median<mode

c) Mean>median>mode   d) None of the above

101. Which of the following is not an input device of a computer

a) Key board   d) Scanner

c) Printer   d) Web camera

102. The test commonly used for comparing the mean of two groups independently drawn from the population is.

a) t- test   b) Z -test

c) P^2 test   d) F- test

103. The binomial distribution tends to the normal distribution as the number of observations (n)

a) Decrease   b) Increase

c) Remain constant   d) Go to infinity

104. Formula for Chi-Square test is

a) $\Sigma (O-E)^2 / E$ b) $\Sigma (O-E)^2 / O$

c) $\Sigma (E-O)^2 / O$ d) $\Sigma (E-O)^2 / E$

105. Which of the following is correct?

a) AM>GM<HM   b) AM<GM<HM

c) GM>AM>HM   d) AM>GM=HM

e) None

106. The most widely used out put device of computer is

a) ALU   b) CPU

c) VDU   d) DPU

107. Blood glucose level was recorded in 30 patients before and after medication. To test whether the medication has got some effect in controlling blood sugar, the most appropriate test is

a) Normal Deviate test   c) t – test

b) F test   d) Chi-square test

108. Chi-square was given by

a) R.A.Fisher
b) Tippatt
c) Gosset
d) Karl-Pearson

109. Two samples of size 160 and 180 are to be tested for their difference of mean, the appropriate test to be applied is

a) Normal Deviate test
b) 't' test
c) F-test
d) None of these
e) Pair't' test

110. Who is referred as the father of the Computer?

a) Abacus
b) Pascal
c) Charles Babbage
d) Joseph Jacquard

111. Mode is

a) Mode = 3 Median – 2 Mean
b) Mean = 3 (Median – Mean)
c) Mean – Mode = 3 Median – 2 Mean

KEY

1. a) Continuous variable
2. c) Positive correlation
3. d) Intercept
4. b) Median
5. b) Program
6. c) Local control
7. c) To
8. c) Variance
9. a) Monitor
10. a) Sample points
11. a) Input
12 c) 1024 MB
13. d) Height
14. b) super computers
15. d) Permutation
16. c) Symmetrical
17. a) Byte
18. d) Chronological classification
19. d) All the above
20. b) Mid value
21. d) Paired t-test
22. b) Moments
23. a) Mhz
24. b) Chi-square test
25. c) Trial
26. a) Histogram
27. c) Hard copy
28. a) 0.25
29. b) ^
30. c) Geographical information system

31. c) Median
32. c) 24
33. c) Mesokurtic
34. c) 50 %
35. a) * / + -
36. d) Chi-square test
37. b) Increasing number of replications
38. c) Fourth
39. a) Median
40. c) Ogive
41. a) AM = Median = Mode
42. a) Skewness
43. d) 95.45%
44. c) Integer variable
45. b) Compiler
46. c) Million operations per second
47. b) Hardwares
48. a) System software
49. c) Nonimpact printer
50. a) Location (central value)
51. a) Mainframe computers
52. d) 0
53. a) Vacuum tubes
54. c) Both a and b
55. b) n-1
56. a) # sign
57. d) Natural languages
58. b) Relational operator
59. b) Softcopy devices
60. d) All the above
61 c) Mutually exclusive
62. a) Dependent
63. a) Biostatistics
64. d) None of the above
65. b) Mode
66. b) ANOVA
67. d) Universe
68. d) All the above
69. c) Poisson
70. d) Independent events
71. a) Francis Galton
72. c) Statistic
73. c) Pen drive
74. a) Positive correlation
75. d) Chi-square test
76. d) NIC
77. c) ALU
78. a) Machine language
79. c) GIGO
80. b) RAM
81 a) COBOL and FORTRAN
82. a) F test
83. b) 25
84. d) Weighted Arithmetic Mean
85. a) Mean = Median
86. a) Zero
87. b) Zero and 100
88. a) Systematic sampling
89. a) Hard disk
90. c) Coefficient of variation
91. a) Coefficient of variation
92. d) All the above
93. c) Fisher
94. c) Array method
95. a) Ogive

96.	d)	Point estimate	97.	c)	Sign test
98.	a)	Start or stop	99.	c)	Variance
100.	b)	Mean<median<mode	101.	c)	Printer
102.	a	Thomson	103.	d	Waldeyer
104.	a	Morgan	105.	e	None
106.	c	VDU	107.	e	Paired t test
108.	d	Karl Pearson	109.	a	Normal Deviate test
110.	c	Charles Babbage	111.	a	Mode = 3 Median – 2 Mean

4. Match the Most Appropriate

SET I

A	B
a. Search engine	1. Statistic
b. RAM	2. Chi-square test
c. QWERTY	3. Coefficient of variation
d. Output device	4. Business
e. Operating system	5. F. Galton
f. Frequency comparison	6. Key board
g. ROM	7. Google
h. Relative measure	8. Non-volatile memory
i. Regression	9. Printer
j. COBOL	10. UNIX
	11. Volatile memory

SET II

A	B
a. Graphic package	1. Start up time
b. Positively skewed	2. James Bernoulli
c. FORTRAN	3. Gosette
d. GUI	4. Charles Babbage
e. Booting	5. Right tailed
f. CUI	6. Corel draw
g. Binomial distribution	7. Procedural language
h. Student t test	8. Correcting errors
i. Father of computer	9. Windows
j. Debugging	10. DOS
	11. Operating system

SET III

A	B
a. ROM	1. Quantitative character
b. MOPS	2. - μto + μ
c. r_{xy}	3. μ
d. Sample mean	4. Non-volatile memory
e. MIPS	5. Qualitative character
f. Milk yield	6. X
g. RAM	7. Traditional computers
h. Population mean	8. 6^2
i. b_{xy}	9. - 1 to + 1
j. Attribute	10. Super computers
	11. Sequential access memory
	12. Volatile memory

SET IV

A	B
a. QWERTY	1. Fourth moment
b. Search engine	2. 0 to a
c. Normal distribution	3. Control statement
d. Binomial distribution	4. Key Board
e. COBOL	5. First moment
f. Branching	6. 0 to n
g. Mean	7. Bell shaped
h. LET	8. Input statement
i. Kurtosis	9. Forward jump
j. Looping	10. Business
	11. Backward jump
	12. Google

SET V

A	B
a. Mean comparison	1. F test
b. Frequency comparison	2. 0 to μ
c. Regression analysis	3. RBD
d. Binomial distribution	4. - μto + μ
e. ANOVA	5. t test
f. Local control	6. Qualitative variable
g. Floppy disk	7. CRD
h. Poisson distribution	8. Sir Francis Galton
i. Normal distribution	9. Chi square
j. Rank correlation analysis	10. Bernoulli
	11. Storage device

SET VI

	A		B
a.	Mean comparison	1.	Statistic
b.	Sample variance	2.	Z - test
c.	Frequency comparison	3.	s^2
d.	Population	4.	Parameter
e.	Large sample	5.	Geometric mean
f.	Population variance	6.	Sturge's rule
g.	Sample	7.	Coefficient of variation
h.	Mathematical average	8.	S
i.	Percentage	9.	Chi-square
j.	Relative measure	10.	S^2
		11.	t-test
		12.	Arithmetic mean

SET VII

	A		B
a.	High level language	1.	MS word
b.	Language translator	2.	GO TO
c.	Presentation	3.	Small circle
d.	Input or output	4.	Interpreter
e.	Search engine	5.	COBOL
f.	Word processor	6.	Power point
g.	Operating system	7.	Parellelogram
h.	Control statement	8.	Google
i.	Low level language	9.	Windows
j.	Hard copy	10.	Print out
		11.	Machine language

SET VIII

	A		B
a.	Regression	1.	R.A. Fisher
b.	Correction coefficient	2.	Gigabyte
c.	Sample size N<30	3.	Karl Pearson
d.	Measures of central tendency	4.	Small Sample
e.	Normal Distribution	5.	Ha
f.	Operating system	6.	DOS
g.	Standard error	7.	Geometric mean
h.	Analysis of variance	8.	Unimodal
i.	Alternative hypothesis	9.	Measure of Reliability
j.	Memory	10.	Galton

KEY

SET I

	A		B
a.	Search engine	7.	Google
b.	RAM	11.	Volatile memory
c.	QWERT	6.	Key board
d.	Output device	9.	Printer
e.	Operating system	10.	UNIX
f.	Frequency comparison	2.	Chi-square test
g.	ROM	8.	Non-volatile memory
h.	Relative measure	3.	Coefficient of variation
i.	Regression	5.	F. Galton
j.	COBOL	4.	Business

SET II

	A		B
a.	Graphic package	6.	Corel draw
b.	Positively skewed	5.	Right tailed
c.	FORTRAN	7.	Procedural language
d.	GUI	9.	Windows
e.	Booting	1.	Startup time
f.	CUI	10.	DOS
g.	Binomial distribution	2.	James Bernoulli
h.	Student t test	3.	Gosette
i.	Father of computers	4.	Charles Babbage
j.	Debugging	8.	Correcting errors

SET III

	A		B
a.	ROM	4.	Non-volatile memory
b.	MOPS	10.	Super computers
c.	rxy	9.	- 1 to + 1
d.	Sample mean	6.	X
e.	MIPS	7.	Traditional computers
f.	Milk yield	1.	Quantitative character
g.	RAM	12.	Volatile memory
h.	Population mean	3.	μ
i.	bxy	2.	$- \mu$ to $+ \mu$
j.	Attribute	5.	Qualitative character

SET IV

	A		B
a.	QWERTY	4.	Key Board
b.	Search engine	12.	Google
c.	Normal distribution	7.	Bell shaped
d.	Binomial distribution	6.	0 to n
e.	COBOL	10.	Business
f.	Branching	9.	Forward jump
g.	Mean	5.	First moment
h.	LET	8.	Input statement
i.	Kurtosis	1.	Fourth moment
j.	Looping	11.	Backward jump

SET V

	A		B
a.	Mean comparison	5.	t test
b.	Frequency comparison	9.	Chi square
c.	Regression analysis	8.	Sir Francis Galton
d.	Binomial distribution	10.	Bernoulli
e.	ANOVA	1.	F test
f.	Local control	3.	RBD
g.	Floppy disk	11.	Storage device
h.	Poisson distribution	2.	0 to μ
i.	Normal distribution	4.	- $\mu$to + μ
j.	Rank correlation analysis	6.	Qualitative variable

SET VI

	A		B
a.	Mean comparison	11.	t-test
b.	Sample variance	10.	S^2
c.	Frequency comparison	9.	Chi-square
d.	Population	4.	Parameter
e.	Large sample	2.	Z - test
f.	Population variance	3.	s^2
g.	Sample	1.	Statistic
h.	Mathematical average	12.	Arithmetic mean
i.	Percentage	5.	Geometric mean
j.	Relative measure	7.	Coefficient of variation

SET VII

	A		B
a.	High level language	5.	COBOL
b.	Language translator	4.	Interpreter
c.	Presentation	6.	Power point
d.	Input or output	7.	Parellelogram
e.	Search engine	8.	Google
f.	Word processor	1.	MS word
g.	Operating system	9.	Windows
h.	Control statement	2.	GO TO
i.	Low level language	11.	Machine language
j.	Hard copy	10.	Print out

SET VIII

	A		B
a.	Regression	10.	Galton
b.	Correction coefficient	3.	Karl Pearson
c.	Sample size N<30	4.	Small Sample
d.	Measures of central tendency	7.	geometric mean
e.	Normal Distribution	8.	Unimodal
f.	Operating system	6.	DOS
g.	Standard error	9.	Measure of Reliability
h.	Analysis of variance	1.	R.A. Fisher
i.	Alternative hypothesis	5.	Ha
j.	Memory	2.	Gigabyte

5. Expand the Following

1. DBMS
2. VIRUS
3. HTML
4. RBD
5. WWW
6. ANOVA
7. LAN
8. CRD
9. BASIC
10. HTTP
11. IP
12. FAO
13. NIC
14. HDD
15. MAN
16. GIS

17. FORTRAN
18. GIGO
19. CPU
20. ALU
21. MIPS
22. MOPS
23. FDD
24. MSDOS
25. DOS
26. ANACOVA
27. ENIAC
28. H_0 & H_1
29. Wi-Fi

KEY

1. DBMS - Data Base Management system
2. VIRUS - Vital Information Resource Under Siege
3. HTML - Hyper Text Markup Language
4. RBD - Randomized Block Design
5. WWW - World Wide Web
6. ANOVA - Analysis of variance
7. LAN - Local Area Network
8. CRD - Completely Randomized Design
9. BASIC - Beginners All Purpose Symbolic Instruction Code
10. HTTP - Hypertext Transfer Protocol
11. IP - Internet Protocol
12. FAO - Food and Agricultural Organization
13. NIC - National Informatic Centre
14. HDD - Hard Disc Drive
15. MAN - Metropolitan Area Network
16. GIS - Geographical information System
17. Fortran - Formula Translator
18. GIGO - Garbage In Garbage Out
19. CPU - Central Processing Unit
20. ALU - Arithmetic and Logic Unit
21. MIPS - Million Instructions Per Second

22. MOPS - Million Operations Per Second
23. FDD - Floppy Disk Drive
24. MSDOS - Microsoft Disk Operating System
25. DOS - Disk Operating System
26. ANACOVA - Analysis of Covariance
27. ENIAC - Electronic Numeric Integrator And Calculator
28. H_0& H_1 - Null hypothesis and alternate hypothesis
29. Wi-Fi - Wireless Fidelity

6. Define the Following

1. Online input devices
2. Correlation
3. Biostatistics
4. Plotters
5. Coefficient of determination
6. Constant
7. Modem
8. Trial and event
9. Syntax
10. Flow chart
11. String variable
12. Standard normal variable
13. Hypothesis
14. Statistical tests
15. Null hypothesis
16. Population
17. Experimental units
18. Sample
19. Variable

20. Trial and event
21. Modem
22. Syntax
23. Randomization
24. Scatter diagram
25. Statistics
26. Ogive
27. Sturge's rule
28. Mean deviation
29. Probability
30. Mutually exclusive events
31. Exhaustive events
32. Coefficient of variation
33. Normal distribution
34. Class interval
35. F test
36. $\times^2$ test
37. Sampling
38. Normal distribution
39. Mode
40. Vital statistics
41. Range
42. Tabulation
43. Geographical classification

7. Differentiate Between the Following

1. RAM and ROM
2. Subdivided and percentage bar diagram
3. General purpose and specific purpose digital computers

4. Classification and tabulation of data
5. Hardware and software
6. Qualitative and quantitative variables
7. Normal and Binomial distributions
8. ED50 and LD50
9. Additive and multiplicative laws of probability
10. LAN and WAN
11. Type I and Type II errors
12. Permutation and combination
13. Census and survey
14. Large sample test and small sample test
15. Chi square test and F test
16. Mean deviation and standard deviation
17. Therapeutic effect and ceiling effect
18. Fertility and fecundity
19. Incidence rate and attack rate.
20. Normal and Binomial distributions
21. Additive and multiplicative laws of probability
22. CRD and RBD
23. Permutation and combination
24. Test statistic and sample statistic
25. Subdivided and percentage bar diagram
26. Parametric and non-parametric tests
27. Qualitative and quantitative variables
28. Skewnessvs Kurtosis
29. Median & Mode
30. AM & GM
31. Standard error & Standard deviation

8. Write Short Notes on the Following

1. Paired t-test
2. Methods of classification of data
3. Flow chart
4. Bioassay
5. Tabulation of data
6. Diagrammatic representation of data
7. Test of hypothesis
8. Online input devices
9. Scatter diagram
10. Determination of quartile deviation for a continuous series of data
11. Regression analysis
12. Impact printers
13. Mainframe computers
14. Skewness
15. Properties of best estimator
16. Paired t-test
17. Bayes theorem
18. Define regression and correlation. What are the different methods of studying correlation?
19. Write in brief on Analysis of Variance. What are the criteria and the steps involved in conducting test of significance?
20. Stages for performing a test of significance
21. Three principles of Experimentation
22. Bioassay
23. Relative potency
24. Types of dose effect relationship
25. Uses of Vital Statistics
26. Regression coefficient

27. Classification of Data
28. Types of Bar diagram
29. Merits of Geometric mean
30. Uses of measures of dispersion
31. Criteria in using binomial distribution
32. Limitations of LET and IN PUT statements
33. Use of computers in veterinary field
34. Machine language
35. RAM and ROM
36. Computer hardware and software.
37. Principles of experimentation
38. Rank correlation
39. Hardcopy and softcopy
40. Peripheral devices
41. Weighted arithmetic mean
42. Paired t-test
43. Determination of quartile deviation for a continuous series of data
44. Chi-square test
45. Bioassay
46. Anatomy of a computer
47. Graphical representation of data
48. Probability
49. Law of probability
50. Coefficient of variation
51. Elements of vital statistics
52. Graphics
53. Use of computers in veterinary hospital
54. Types of memories
55. The mode of inheritance of sex

56. Variance
57. Parallel line assay
58. Floppies
59. Input and output devices
60. Experimental error
61. F test
62. LD50 and ED50
63. RAM and ROM
64. Mean and Median
65. Therapeutic index
66. Regression curve
67. Test of significance
68. Computer languages
69. Kurtosis
70. Properties of best estimator
71. Chi-square test for goodness of fit
72. Classification of computers based on operating principles
73. Explain CPU
74. Describe major applications of computer
75. The properties of T- test.
76. Normal distribution with its Properties.
77. Define completely randomized design with advantage and disadvantage
78. Write down/ prepare flow chart
79. Write down properties of regression co-efficient

9. Write Essay on the Following

1. a. What is a computer? Indicate the main components of a personal computer.

   b. List out the input and output devices that are necessary in daily computer operations.

c. What is the importance of computer application in the field of Veterinary and Animal Sciences?

2. a. What is an experimental design and how it is useful in the field of animal sciences.

   b. Explain the basic principles of experimentation

   c. Briefly describe the difference between one way and two way analysis of variance.

3. a. What is correlation? Describe the method of estimation of Karl Pearson's correlation coefficient.

   b. What is regression analysis? Describe the difference between correlation and regression analysis

4. a. Define measures of central tendency

   b. Describe the different measures of central tendency

   c. Elaborate the methods of calculation of positional averages for different types of data with their advantage and disadvantages.

5. a. Define and discuss in detail about GIS.

   b. Discuss the NIC

   c. Explain in detail the use of computers in farm, statistical analysis and epidemiology

6. a. What is a computer? Indicate the main components of a PC or digital computer.

   b. List out the input and output devices that are necessary in daily computer operations.

   c. What is the importance of computer applications in Veterinary and Animal Sciences

7. What is a non-parametric test.Describe the chi-square test for goodness of fit and test of independence. Describe the application of chi-square test with an example

8. Explain in detail the procedure of randomized block design with example

9. a. What is a computer? What are its components, explain them briefly

   b. Explain crude death rate, age specific fertility rate

10. a. Define a statistical hypothesis

    b. Differentiate between null and alternate hypothesis

    c. What do you understand by level of significance

11. a. Enumerate the measures of central tendency and explain about each of them

    b. List and detail the steps in developing a computer program. Write a program in BASIC to calculate the mean for 4 number of observations

12. a. What is type I and type II errors and level of significance in testing of hypothesis.

    b. Give procedure for testing the hypothesis

    c. Describe different measures of dispersion

    d. Define correlation. Write down different formulae used in its calculation

    e. What is computer and discuss its component

    f. Differentiate between hardware and software

13. a. What is randomized block design

    b. Explain the procedure of analysis for RBD

    c. Give merits and demerits of RBD over CRD

    d. Explain different types of computers

14. What is frequency and frequency distribution? Write general principles of frequency distribution.

    b. Explain dose-response relationship

    c. Differentiate between continuous and discrete variables

15. a. What is meant by t-test of significance?

    b. Discuss the Randomized block design

    c. Explain use of computer for statistical analysis

16. What do you understand by measure of central tendency? Mention their names and explain any two methods along with procedures.

    What is a computer? Discuss its various components.

17. a. Define statistics. What are its importance

    b. Define histogram &frequency curve

    c. Explain continuous frequency distribution

18. a. Explain completely randomized design

    b. Explain the basic principles of experimental design

19. a. Write the properties of normal distribution

    b. Define and give a formula for mean, median and mode

    c. What are the application of t-test

20. a. What are computers? Discuss its various components

    b. What is frequency and frequency distribution? Write general principles of frequency distribution

    c. Explain dose-response relationship

21. a. Define sampling and specify its objective

    b. Enumerate the methods of sampling

    c. How random sampling is advantageous over other methods of sampling?

22. a. What is bioassay? How will you proceed in conducting bioassay of a drug?

    b. What are vital statistics? How do you estimate the mortality rate in animals due to outbreak of rinderpest disease?

23. a. Describes different types of computers.

    b. Discuss in detail the use of information technology in animal health

24. Explain the concept of design of experiments. Differentiate between CRD and RBD with respect to their principles and procedures.

❑❑❑

AGB-121 : PRINCIPLES OF ANIMAL GENETICS AND POPULATION GENETICS

Section-II

AGB 121 Principles of Animal Genetics and Population Genetics

1. Fill in the Blanks with the Most Suitable Answer

1. Inter-allelic interaction is known as ____________________
2. The classical 9:3:3:1 ratio becomes _____________ in case of dominant epistasis
3. Genes on Y chromosome are designated as ___________________
4. Total phenotypic variance is partitioned into _______________ and _______________
5. If the frequency of gene 'A' is 0.3, then the genotype frequency of AA individuals is ________________
6. In ABO blood group system, genotype of 'O' group is _____________
7. The individual with identical sex chromosome is termed as _________________
8. Mutation from A to T is known as ______________ and from T to C is known as ________________
9. If the dominant allele of one locus and the recessive allele of the other occupy the same chromosome (Ab/aB) the linkage is called ___________________ phase
10. Change in one or few chromosome is termed as _______________
11. A series of three or more forms of a gene in a locus is termed as _________________

12. Arrangement of chromosomes based on length and position of centromere is termed as ______________
13. A trait which is expressed in only one sex is termed as ______________
14. Mutations occurring in non-reproductive cells are called ______________
15. Phenotypic variance is made up of genotypic variance and ______________ variance
16. Sperm of a boar has ______________ number of chromosomes
17. Germplasm theory was proposed by ______________
18. ______________ method of heritability estimation is more reliable in cattle
19. ______________ is an important tool to change the gene frequencies in a desired direction
20. ______________ is father of genetics
21. The word gene was first coined by ______________
22. The two fundamental laws of heredity are ______________ and ______________
23. Heritability ranges from ______________ and ______________
24. V_A/V_P is heritability in ______________ sense.
25. Sudden heritable change in the structure of gene is known as ______________
26. The forces that may change the gene frequency are ______________, ______________ and ______________
27. ABO blood group system in human being is an example for ______________ inheritance
28. Phenotypic ratio of F_2dihybrid cross is ______________
29. The probability of getting homozygous dominant offspring from two heterozygote parent is ______________
30. Expression of two alleles in a heterozygote that produce a phenotype to be distinguished from either of its homozygotes is termed as ______________
31. The cell division in which the number of chromosomes is reduced to half is known as ______________

32. Full word of DNA is ____________________________
33. The encasement theory was proposed by _____________
34. __________________ developed the preformation theory
35. The autosomal allele that is expressed only when it is in homozygous condition is termed ____________________
36. A pyrimidine base found in both DNA and RNA is ______________
37. The failure of chromosome to separate in mitosis or meiosis is referred as ____________________
38. Turner syndrome is found in woman who have _________________ sex chromosome composition
39. The principle enzyme that catalyzes the DNA replication is ______________________
40. The genes that can move from one genetic element or chromosome to other are known as ___________________.
41. The DNA replication occurs in the _____________ phase of cell cycle
42. ______________ first demonstrated the mutagenic effect of X-rays through ClB technique
43. The chromosome number of sheep is ________________ and that of goat is ___________________
44. Congenital hyperuricemia characterized by the production of excess uric acid is inherited through a _________________
45. The marriage of Rh+ve father and Rh-ve mother may cause a condition called ________________ in the progenies
46. Haemophilia in human being is a condition to bleed freely is inherited by ________________ gene
47. The forces which changes gene frequency in a small population are ____________________ and _________________
48. In case of recessive epistasis the phenotypic ratio is _______________
49. A polyploidy having chromosome set of two different species is called _______________
50. Reappearance of remote ancestral traits is known as ________________
51. Mendel presented his work in the meeting of National History Society of Brunn in the year _____________

52. The vapour theory of inheritance was proposed by __________
53. The phenotypic ratio in dominant and recessive epistasis is __________
54. The number of different kinds of gametes formed by the F_1 hybrid can be calculated by the formula ____________
55. The branch of biology which deals with the chromosomes and their implication in genetics is known as ______________
56. The enzyme that joins the ends of two strands of nucleic acid is ________________
57. The ratio of X-chromosome number and number of sets of autosomes for intersex is between _______________
58. Extra chromosomal DNA molecules that replicate independently and maintain themselves in the cytoplasm of cells are called ________________
59. The scientist ________________________ proposed that some human diseases are due to inborn errors of metabolism that result from the lack of specific enzyme.
60. Sperm of rabbit has ______________ number of chromosomes
61. Two main aspects of genetic mapping are _________________ and ________________
62. Transformation experiment in mice was studied by ______________
63. Barred plumage in birds is an example for _________________ trait
64. The maximum crossing over percentage would be ______________
65. The possible genotypes of Himalayan rabbits are _______________ and ________________
66. A complete set of genes inherited as a unit from one parent is called ________________
67. A gene causing the death of an organism before or after its birth is termed as ________________
68. A female calf born co-twin to a male, having abnormal reproductive character is called ______________
69. Normal chromosome number in the kidney cell of a sheep is __________
70. The tRNA carries the ________________ to bring in the specific amino acid required for protein synthesis at the ribosomes

71. Sex linked genes are carried only on ______________ chromosome
72. ______________ traits expresses differently in different sexes in heterozygous condition
73. Mutation which occurs in sex cell is known as ____________
74. No. of eggs produced from six primary oocytes are ______________
75. Mating of F_1 individual with any one of the parental type is known as ______________
76. The total genes possessed by males and females of a population is called as ______________
77. Repeatability is generally estimated by ______________ method
78. In an idealized population, the initial random mating population is referred as ______________ and the sub populations are referred as ______________
79. The genetic constitution of the population is expressed in terms of ____________ and ____________
80. Three important genetic parameters are ________________, ________________ and ________________
81. The terms phenotype and genotype were proposed by ____________
82. Intra allelic interaction is known as _____________
83. The noncoding regions of eukaryotic genes are known as __________
84. The co-dominance and incomplete dominance are modifications of ____________ ratios
85. An example for sex influenced trait in Ayrshire cattle is ___________
86. The process in which a polypeptide chain is synthesized in the ribosome in accordance with the codon sequence of a mRNA is known as ____________
87. Coding regions of eukaryotic genes are designated as ______________
88. The longest phase of cell cycle is ____________
89. The mutagenic effect of mustard gas is due to ______________
90. The maximum possible F_2 genotypes in a typical tetra hybrid cross is ____________
91. Genes of the same chromosome which do not assort independently are designated as ____________

92. The phenomenon of genes located on the same chromosome tend to remain together during sexual reproduction is called ____________

93. In chicken when two creepers are mated, the phenotypic ratio of the progeny generation will be ____________

94. Mating of F_1hybrid with the homozygous recessive parent is known as ____________

95. In a population under Hardy Weinberg equilibrium, if the gene frequency of A_1 and A_2 alleles are 0.6 and 0.4 respectively, the genotype frequency of A_1A_2 would be ____________

96. Exchange of segments between two non-homologous chromosomes is known as ____________

97. The ratio of genetic variance to the total phenotypic variance is termed as ____________

98. The process of formation of mRNA from DNA is known as ____________

99. The monohybrid genotypic ratio is ____________

100. The theories of "Use and disuse of organs" and "Inheritance of acquired characters" were proposed by ____________

101. When both alleles of a pair are fully expressed in a heterozygote, they are called ____________

102. The value of an individual judged by the mean value of its progenies is called as ____________

103. In recombinant DNA technology the enzymes used to cut the DNA are called as ____________

104. Random fluctuations in gene frequency in small population is known as ____________

105. The contribution of offspring to the next generation is called ____________ of an individual.

106. Indirect selection will be effective only when the genetic correlation between two traits considered is ____________

107. A chromosome in which centromere is at the centre is called ____________

108. The mutation caused by the substitution of one purine by another purine is termed as ____________

109. Presence of three or more sets of chromosomes is called ____________

110. The unit containing complete set of genes inherited from one parent is ________________

111. The number of hydrogen bonds between G and C are ____________

112. Criss-cross pattern of inheritance is a characteristic feature of ___________ inheritance

113. Bridges proposed the ____________ method of sex determination

114. The chain initiating codon is ______________

115. Mutations occurring in non-reproductive cell is termed as _______________

116. Individuals with identical sex chromosomes are called _________________

117. If p = 0.5, the number of heterozygote individuals in a population of 1000 will be ___________________

118. Suppression of a gene pair at one locus by a gene pair at another locus is termed as ______________

119. The modified dihybrid ratio in duplicate dominant epistasis is _____________

120. A sheep ovum contains ________________ number of chromosomes

121. Haemophilia in man and pigs is a ____________ trait

122. Chromosome number in any species over generations is maintained through __________________

123. If the dominant allele of one locus and the recessive allele of the other locus are present on the same chromosome, the relationship is termed as ________________ phase

124. Number of a particular gene occurring in a population is expressed in terms of _________________

125. The condition wherein only one gene brings about the expression of a character is termed as _________________

126. The genes located on the Y chromosome are termed as ____________

127. Mutations occurring in non-reproductive cells are called as _____________ mutation

128. The alternative form of a gene is known as ______________

129. The possible genotypes of A blood group in human are ____________ and ________________

130. ____________ is an exception to Mendel's principle of random assortment.

131. The horn pattern in Dorset sheep is an example for ________________ inheritance

132. A cross between parents differing in only one trait or in which only one trait is being considered is called ______________

133. The ______________ and ______________ are the reasons for genetic correlation between two or more traits

134. The theory of epigenesis was proposed by ________________

135. Xanthine is deaminated product of ____________

136. Total number of barr bodies in an individual with Turner's syndrome is ____________

137. If a woman heterozygous for colour blindness marries a colour blind man, the probability that their first child will be colour blind daughter is ___________

138. Shortest phase in mitosis is __________

139. Soluble RNA (sRNA) is _____________

140. The number of linkage group in swamp buffalo is ______________

141. Total number of genotypes in human ABO blood group system is ____________

142. Histone proteins are basic because they contain 20-30 per cent ____________ and _____________ positively charged amino acids

143. The deeply staining areas of chromatin material that remain condensed even in metaphase nucleus is called ________________

144. The monohybrid phenotypic ratio is ________________

145. The location of a gene on a chromosome is called ________________

146. Genetics is the branch of science which deals with the study of ______________ and ___________________

147. Egg production in chicken is a sex ____________ trait

148. Linkage is an exception to the law of _________________ and _________________ is an exception to linkage

149. Heritability is the regression of breeding value on _______________ value

150. The phenomena of final maturation of the spermatids into spermatozoa is called _________________

151. ____________________ is the terminology used to describe the process where sex of the offspring is determined before fertilization and _______________ is the terminology for sex determination at the time of fertilization

152. The repetition of the same trait several times during the lifetime of the same individual is measured as _____________________

153. The fitness of an individual that dies before the age of reproduction is _____________

154. __________________ is the raw material for selection

155. The concept of ________________ indicates the regression of the future performance on the past records

156. ________________ is one of the major milestones in the history of genetics launched with an objective to map and sequence all human genes

157. The inheritance of traits controlled by the genes of mother but expressed in the progeny are called as _________________

158. Five different phases of meiotic prophase are _______________, ______________, _______________, _____________ and _____________

159. When a locus contains 3 alleles in a population, the number of heterozygotes would be _______________ out of a total of _____________ number of genotypes

160. The magnitude of genetic drift is larger when the population size is ________________

161. _______________ is a sex-influenced traits in human being where as _______________is a sex limited trait in cattle.

162. The dispersive force that changes gene frequency is _______________.

163. The chromosomal aberration where there is exchange of the part of non-Chromosome is called as _________________.

164. Genetic properties of a population are expressible in terms of the __________ and _______________________ frequencies.

165. ____________ refers to interallelic interaction.

166. ____________ is the father of modern theory of evolution.

167. Snail coiling is an example of ____________ whereas the variegation of the leaves of 4 'O' clock plant is an example of ______________.

168. The term genetics was coined by ______________________

169. The process of exchange of portion between two non-sistered homologous chromosome is called_____________________________

170. A monohybrid is _________________for one pair of allelic gene

171. An individual producing only one type of gamete is known as__________________

172. In ___________ phase of cell division chiasmata formation takes place

173. The father of a colour blind girl will be _______________________

174. Male transmit his __________________gene to his grandsons through his daughter

175. ________________ is the transfer of genetic materials from one genotype to another by bacteriophase

176. _________________ mutations are not transmitted to the progeny

177. The diploid no of chromosome in swamp buffalo is ____________.

KEY

1. Epistasis
2. 12:3:1
3. Holandric genes
4. Genotypic and environmental
5. 0.09
6. I^oI^o
7. Homogametic
8. Transversion, Transition
9. Repulsion
10. Aneuploidy
11. Multiple alleles
12. Karyotyping
13. Sex limited
14. Somatic mutations
15. Environmental variance
16. 19
17. August Weissman
18. Half sib
19. Selection
20. Gregor Johann Mendel
21. Johannsen
22. Law of segregation and law of random assortment

23. Zero and one
24. Narrow
25. Mutation
26. Migration, mutation and selection
27. Multiple alleles
28. 9:3:3:1
29. 25% or ¼
30. Incomplete dominance
31. Meiosis
32. Deoxyribonucleic acid
33. Charles Bonnet
34. Jan Swammerdam
35. Recessive
36. Cytosine
37. Nondisjunction
38. 45 X
39. DNA polymerase
40. Transposons or jumping genes
41. Synthetic
42. H.J. Muller
43. 54,60
44. Sex linked recessive
45. Erythroblastosisfetalis
46. Sex linked recessive gene
47. Genetic drift and inbreeding
48. 9:3:4
49. Allopolyploid
50. Atavism
51. 1865
52. Pythagoras
53. 13:3
54. 2^n
55. Cytogenetics
56. Ligase
57. 0.5 and 1.0
58. Plasmids
59. ArchibalfdGarrod
60. 22
61. Gene order and gene distance
62. Griffith
63. Sex linked
64. 50
65. $c^hc^h$and c^hc
66. Genome
67. Lethal Gene
68. Freemartin
69. 54
70. Anticodon
71. X chromosome
72. Sex influenced
73. Germinal mutation
74. Six
75. Back crossing
76. Gene pool
77. Intra class correlation
78. Base population, lines
79. Gene and Genotype frequencies
80. Heritability, repeatability and genetic correlation
81. Johannson
82. Dominance
83. Introns
84. Monohybrid

85. Coat color
86. Translation
87. Exons
88. Interphase
89. Alkylation of bases
90. $(3)^4$ or 81
91. Linked
92. Linkage
93. 1:2, Normal: Creeper
94. Test cross
95. 0.48
96. Translocation
97. Heritability in broad sense
98. Transcription
99. 1:2:1
100. Lamarck
101. co-dominant
102. breeding value
103. Restriction enzymes
104. Random drift/ Genetic drift
105. Fitness/ adoptive value/ selective value
106. High
107. Metacentric
108. Transition
109. Polyploidy
110. Gamete
111. Three
112. Sex-linked
113. Genic balance
114. AUG
115. Somatic cell
116. Homogametic
117. 500
118. Epistasis
119. 15:1
120. 27
121. Sex-linked
122. Meiosis
123. Repulsion/Trans
124. Gene frequency
125. Pseudominance
126. Holandric genes
127. Somatic cell
128. Allele
129. $I^AI^A$and I^AI^O
130. Epistasis
131. Sex-linked
132. Monohybrid cross
133. Pleiotropy and linkage
134. K.F. Wolff
135. Guanine
136. Zero
137. 25%
138. Anaphase
139. tRNA
140. 24
141. 6
142. Arginine and lysine
143. Heterochromatin
144. 3:1
145. Locus
146. Heredity and variation
147. Sex limited
148. Random assortment, crossing over

149. Phenotypic value
150. Spermatogenesis
151. Progameic and syngamic
152. Repeatability
153. Zero
154. Variation
155. Repeatability
156. Human genome project
157. Maternal inheritance
158. Leptotene, zygotene, pachytene, diplotene and diakinesis
159. 3, 6
160. Small
161. Baldness milk yield
162. Random drift
163. Reciprocal translocation
164. Gene genotype
165. Epistasis
166. Darwin
167. Cytoplasmicinheritance Cytoplasmic inheritance
168. Bateson
169. Crossing over
170. Heterozygotes
171. Homogematic
172. Pachytene
173. Colourblind
174. Sexlinked
175. Transduction
176. Somatic
177. 48

2. True or False

1. Quantitative traits are governed by major genes and environment has little or no effect on the expression of these traits
2. The phenomenon in which one gene influences the expression of several characters is termed pleiotropy
3. In panmictic population, some animals are more preferred over others in a breeding programme
4. Heterochromatins are the lightly staining regions of the chromosomes.
5. Only two alleles are sufficient for the expression of a trait in multiple allelic series
6. The frequency of a heterozygote will be maximum when the gene frequency of the alleles at a locus are equal
7. Mutation provides the raw material for selection
8. The heritability sets the upper limit of repeatability
9. Reverse mutation is more common than forward mutation
10. DNA structure was first explained by Mendel

11. The heritability in broad sense is more reliable than the heritability in narrow sense
12. Crossing over increases with increase in the distance between genes
13. In meiosis, each daughter cell will have identical number of chromosomes as that of parents
14. A gene that appears to produce its effect only in homozygous condition has recessive gene action
15. The noncoding regions of eukaryotic genes are known as exons
16. An individual who carries a recessive gene that is not expressed is called carrier
17. UGA is a start codon
18. Genes of both sex linked and sex influenced traits are located on the sex chromosomes
19. Generally quantitative characters in livestock have no economic importance
20. Milk production is a sex limited trait and hence bulls do not carry the genes for it
21. The repeatability estimate for birth weight in calves is always high
22. Mutations may occur at any stage in the life of an individual or organism and different genes have different rates of mutation
23. The genes carried by the population have continuity from generation to generation, but genotypes in which they appear do not
24. Watson and Crick got Nobel prize for the discovery of double helix structure of DNA
25. The test of choice for studying the Hardy-Weinberg equilibrium in a population is chi-square test.
26. The genes are arranged in a linear fashion on the chromosomes
27. Iso-chromosome is a metacentric chromosome in which the two arms are structurally and genetically identical
28. The Turner's syndrome is seen in males with a chromosomal complement of 47, XXY
29. Most probable producing ability is mostly estimated to select the bulls rather than to select the cows

30. In pericentric inversions, the centromere is included within the inverted sequence
31. Chi-square test is to be used for testing the population whether it is in Hardy-Weinberg equilibrium or not
32. The rate of reverse ' is higher than forward mutation
33. 65, XXY in horse is equivalent to the Klinefelter's syndrome in man
34. Cryptorchidism is a sex linked trait
35. Gene pool is defined as the sum of all genotypes present in a given population
36. One gene-one enzyme hypothesis was proposed by Beadle and Tatum
37. Tortoise shell condition in cats is due to co-dominant sex linked genes
38. The phenomenon in which more traits are influenced by one gene is termed as pleiotropy
39. Sickle cell anemia is due to point mutation, in which the glutamic acid is replaced by valine
40. Freemartin could be of either sex
41. Quantitative characters have no economic importance
42. Epistasis is the interaction between non allelic genes
43. The number of ovum resulting from 6 primary oocytes is 12
44. Barred plumage in poultry is an example of sex linked trait
45. AB x AB blood group parents cannot produce 'A' blood group offspring
46. If the dominant gene frequency is 0.8, the homozygous recessive genotype frequency is 0.04
47. The sex of drosophila flies with a sex index of 0.50 is male
48. Synthesis of mRNA from DNA is termed as transcription
49. Gene frequency ranges between 1 to 2
50. Except for sperm, all other cells of a bull have 60, XY chromosome complement
51. Environmental variations reduce the accuracy of selection in genetic studies
52. Test crossing and back crossing are same

53. When heritability of a trait is more, the accuracy of individual selection is more
54. Non-additive variance is the main cause of resemblance between relatives
55. Independent assortment of law of heredity holds universally
56. If the repeated measures of the same animal are similar to each other, the trait is said to be lowly repeatable
57. Down's syndrome individuals are trisomic of sex chromosome
58. In complete dominance the phenotype of heterozygotes will be different from both homozygotes
59. Exchange of genetic material between non homologous chromosome is known as translocation
60. Sex limited genes present only in sex chromosomes
61. Genetic variability within a population is necessary if selection is said to be effective over a long period of time
62. Uracil is present in RNA molecule
63. Quantitative traits are not influenced by environmental factors
64. Additive genetic value and breeding value of an individual are different
65. Chromosome number of trisomic can be represented as 2n+1
66. Migration is the strongest force for changing the gene frequency
67. Relationship between full sibs is 0.5
68. Heritability ranges between 0 and 1
69. Thymine is a pyrimidine base
70. The number of chromosome in bull spermatozoa is 60
71. It is possible to get all possible blood groups if the parents are of AB and A blood group
72. The genes carried on the Y chromosome are called holandric genes
73. Traits with low heritability can be improved by altering the management
74. In a random mating population, maximum heterozygosity is expressed when the gene frequency is 0.2
75. If a trait is largely controlled by environment, the heritability would be very high

76. Semi-lethal genes cause death of an individual before birth or at birth itself
77. Heterochromatin are darkly stained regions of chromosomes
78. In a litter of 6 piglets, the chances of obtaining 3 males and 3 females are 20/64
79. Independent assortment is applicable to genes present on different chromosomes
80. Recombination of linked genes is accomplished by crossing over
81. The appearance of more numbers of parental types in a test than recombinant type is indicative of linkage
82. Change in entire set of chromosome number is termed euploidy
83. Two main aspects of genetic mapping are gene order and gene distance
84. In a panmictic population, some animals are preferred over others in a breeding programme
85. In repulsion phase, two dominant or two recessive genes will be present on the same chromosomes
86. Generally speaking the full sib correlation and regression of offspring on dam are the most reliable methods to estimate heritability in cattle
87. A crossing between F_1 hybrid with homozygous recessive individual is known as parent cross
88. Qualitative traits are discontinuous and can be classified into distinct classes
89. Nonexistence of 9:3:3:1 phenotypic ratio in F_2 could be an indication of epistatic interaction
90. Aneuploidy refers to at least one more or one less chromosome than the diploid number.
91. Milk production is a sex limited trait and hence selection of bulls do not improve the milk yield in subsequent generations
92. In a normal human male cell, there will be no Barr bodies
93. Litter size at birth in swine is highly heritable trait
94. Heritability indicates the reliability of the early performance records as a guide to predict future performance
95. The full sib correlation method gives the upper limit of heritability

96. The milk yield in cattle is a medium heritable trait

97. Regression of breeding value on phenotypic value is heritability

98. Breeding value represents part of genotypic value that can be transmitted from parent to offspring

99. Quantitative traits are governed by one or a few pairs of genes and environment has little or no effect on the expression of these traits

100. The major cause of genetic correlation is linkage and pleiotropy of genes

101. Heritability estimates give a measure of the accuracy with which selection for a genotype can be made from phenotype of the individual

102. Heritability estimates of traits like conception rate, early viability and litter size are high

103. When heritability of a trait is low, it can be inferred that the trait is mostly influenced by the environment and selection of sire would bring minimum response

104. If the frequency of dominant gene is 0.8 then the frequency of recessive gene will be 0.7

105. In a random mating population some animals are preferred over other animals in a breeding programme.

106. Heritability estimate for a particular trait is lower than repeatability as the later contains the environment component also.

107. Degree of resemblance between relatives is the basis of different methods of heritability estimation.

108. The repeatability estimate of birth weight in calves is 0.25

109. In a litter of 5 piglets, the probability of obtaining all females is 1/32

110. Genes located on the same chromosome assort independently irrespective of the distance between them

111. In co-dominance, the heterozygotes are similar to both parental genotypes

112. When the frequency of recessive gene is 0.5, then half of the population will have the dominant character

113. Chromosome theory of linkage was proposed by Sutton and Bovery

114. In half sib analysis, the covariance between sire estimates one half of the covariance of the breeding values of the two traits

115. Gene frequency is the number of genes present in the population

116. Panmixia does not affect the gene frequency
117. Walnut comb in chicken is due to complementary interaction of genes at a single locus
118. Inversion causes apparent loss of genetic material in the chromosome
119. All genes responsible for sex-limited inheritance are located on sex chromosomes
120. Diagrammatic representation of the chromosome is called ideogram
121. The colour blindness in human being is an example for sex linked recessive gene action
122. The phenomenon of genes located on the same chromosome tend to remain together during sexual reproduction is called isochromosomes
123. In chicken when two creepers are mated, the phenotypic ratio of the progeny generation will be 3:1
124. Adenine is pyrimidine base found both in DNA and RNA
125. The chromosome that has its centromere near the end is called acrosome
126. Chromosome fragment lacking a centromere is known as acentric chromosome
127. A polyploidy that has multiple and identical sets of chromosomes derived from the same species are known as autopolyploid
128. Any chromosome that is not a sex chromosome is called as autosomes
129. The process by which chromosomes exchange genetic material through the breakage and reunion of their DNA molecules is called Crossing over
130. The degree of expression of a trait controlled by a gene is known as expressivity
131. The proportion of population that suffers genetic death is called genetic load
132. The Hardy-Weinberg law holds good for both large and small populations
133. Intersex is an organism displaying secondary sexual character intermediate between male and female
134. The nuclear gene k is required for maintenance of kappa in the cytoplasm of killer strains of *Paramecium aurelia*

135. The stage of cell division in which the chromosomes are most discrete and arranged in an equatorial plate is called metaphase

136. An environmental agent, either physical or chemical that is capable of inducing mutations are known as mutagen

137. The condition in which the heterozygote is superior to both the homozygotes is known as over dominance

138. The observable characteristics of an organism is called phenocopy

139. The branch of science that deals with the genetic constitution of the population is known as population genetics

140. The process of formation of sperm from spermatids is called Spermiogenesis

141. In case of sex limited inheritance the gene responsible is located on the X chromosome

142. The maximum number of linkage groups possible in an organism is equal to the number of pairs of chromosomes present in the diploid cell.

143. Inheritance of snail coiling pattern is an example of maternal effect.

144. The phenotypic ration observed in a cross of double heterozygote in duplicate dominant epistasis is 9 : 7.

145. Psedodominance is a condition which is observed when there is structural chromosomal anomaly.

146. Deaf – Mute condition in human being is an example of dominant epistatis.

147. There is no dominance – recessive relation between the alleles when there is co-dominance.

148. Erythroblastosisfetalis is a physiological disorder due to lack of secretion of Erythropiotin in humans.

149. Average effect is a property of gene and genotype.

150. Selection does not change gene frequency of random mating population

151. Colour blindness is a sex-limited trait

152. Sex- influenced inheritance follows a Zig-Zag pattern

153. Mammalian females are hetero gametic sex

154. Females of poultry are heterogametic sex

155. Presence of horns/polled condition is a quantative trait
156. Mendalian genetics can not be extended to quantitative genetics
157. Half sibs are the individuals born by the same dam mated to different sires
158. A single generation of random mating brings the gene frequency to H-W equilibrium in the population
159. If the gene frequency of a lethal gene is very high in a population it takes many generations to eliminate the gene from the population
160. Percentage of the individuals expressing the phenotype due to the presence of gene is called as the penetrance of the gene in the population

KEY

1.	False	2.	True
3.	False	4.	False
5.	True	6.	True
7.	True	8.	False
9.	False	10.	False
11.	False	12.	True
13.	False	14.	True
15.	False	16.	True
17.	False	18.	False
19.	False	20.	False
21.	False	22.	True
23.	True	24.	True
25.	True	26.	True
27.	True	28.	False
29.	False	30.	True
31.	True	32.	False
33.	True	34.	True
35.	False	36.	True
37.	False	38.	True
39.	True	40.	False
41.	False	42.	True
43.	False	44.	True

45. False
46. True
47. True
48. True
49. False
50. True
51. True
52. False
53. True
54. False
55. True
56. False
57. False
58. False
59. True
60. False
61. True
62. True
63. False
64. False
65. True
66. True
67. True
68. True
69. True
70. False
71. False
72. True
73. True
74. False
75. False
76. False
77. True
78. True
79. True
80. True
81. True
82. True
83. True
84. False
85. False
86. False
87. False
88. True
89. True
90. True
91. False
92. True
93. False
94. False
95. True
96. True
97. True
98. True
99. False
100. True
101. True
102. False
103. True
104. False
105. False
106. True
107. True
108. False
109. True
110. False
111. False
112. False

113. True
114. False
115. False
116. True
117. False
118. False
119. False
120. True
121. True
122. False
123. False
124. False
125. False
126. True
127. True
128. True
129. True
130. True
131. True
132. False
133. True
134. True
135. True
136. True
137. True
138. False
139. True
140. True
141. False
142. False
143. False
144. False
145. True
146. False
147. True
148. False
149. False
150. False
151. False
152. False
153. False
154. True
155. False
156. True
157. True
158. True
159. False
160. True

3. Choose the Most Appropriate Answer

1. Number of sex chromosomes present in a spermatozoa

   a) One
   b) Two
   c) Nil
   d) 23

2. The ultimate source of all genetic variation which provides raw materials for evolution is

   a) Pleiotropy
   b) Breeding
   c) Mutation
   d) Linkage

3. Hen is a

   a. Homogametic　　b. Heterogametic

   c. Isogametic　　d. None of the above

4. The metacentric chromosome having two structurally and genetically identical arms are termed as

   a. Ring chromosomes　　b Similar chromosomes

   c. Isochromosome　　d. None of the above

5. The cell division stage, most ideal for chromosome study is

   a. Telophase　　b. Metaphase

   c. Anaphase　　d. None of the above

6. The chromosal configuration of a domestic ram is

   a. 52, XX　　b. 54, XY

   c. 60, XY　　d. 58, XY

7. The theory of pangenesis was proposed by

   a. Charles Darwin　　b. Spallanzani

   c. Lamark　　d. Mendel

8. Which of the following blood groups cannot be that of father of a child with blood group O, born to a woman with a blood group A?

   a. Man with blood group A　　b. Man with blood group B

   c. Man with blood group AB　　d. Man with blood group O

9. The diploid chromosome number of horse is

   a. 82　　b. 72

   c. 64　　d. 88

10. The following F_2 phenotypic ratio is not an indication of epistasis interaction

    a. 12:3:1　　b. 9:7

    c. 9:6:1　　d. 9:3:3:1

11. Hair on ear pinna is an example of

    a. Recessive epistasis　　b. Codominance

    c. Holandric inheritance　　d. Linkage

12. Interchange of individuals between populations is known as
    a. Mutation b. Selection
    c. Migration d. Random drift

13. The chromosome number of a person suffering from Klinefelter's syndrome is
    a. 45 b. 46
    c. 48 d. 47

14. The following F_2 phenotypic ratio is not an indication of epistasis
    a. 12:3:1 b. 9:7
    c. 1:2:1 d. 9:6:1

15. The MN blood group is controlled by the gene action
    a. Co-dominant b. Multiple alleles
    c. Polygenes d. Cytoplasmic inheritance

16. Chiasma frequency between any two genetic loci is directly proportional to the
    a. Distance between them b. Number of genes
    c. Both the above d. None of the above

17. The number of sperms resulting from 6 primary spermatocytes is
    a. 6 b. 12
    c. 18 d. 24

18. The mating of F_1 individual with any one of the parental type is
    a. Inter se mating b. Test cross
    c. Back cross d. Grading up

19. Polyploidy can be created artificially by treatment with
    a. Mustard gas b. Colchicine
    c. Giemsa d. None of the above

20. Criss-cross pattern of inheritance is the characteristic feature of
    a. Sex linked traits b. Sex influenced traits
    c. Sex limited traits d. None of the above

21. Holandric traits are passed on from father to
    a. Son only
    b. Daughters only
    c. Both Sons and daughters
    d. Only to grand daughters
22. Genes for milk production are present in
    a. Males only
    b. Females only
    c. Both males and females
    d. Only in bulls
23. Germplasm theory of inheritance was proposed by
    a. Weissmann
    b. Darwin
    c. Lamark
    d. None of the above
24. Individuals with Klinefelter's syndrome are sex chromatin
    a. Positive
    b. Negative
    c. Either of the two
    d. None of the above
25. Crossing over is absent in drosophila
    a. Females
    b. Males
    c. Neither
    d. Both the above
26. Walnut type of comb in chicken results from crossing of
    a. Single X Rose
    b. Single x Pea
    c. Pea X Pea
    d. Rose X Pea
27. Law of Segregation is also known as
    a. Law of impurity of gametes
    b. Law of purity of gametes
    c. Law of improbability
    d. Law of random assortment
28. In chicken heterogametic sex is
    a. Male
    b. Female
    c. None of the above
    d. Both male and female
29. 13:3 is the ratio of
    a. Dominant & recessive epistasis
    b. Duplicate dominant epistasis
    c. Duplicate recessive epistasis
    d. None of the above

30. The concept of Genotype and Phenotype was introduced by

a. W. Johanssen
b. Fisher
c. William Bateson
d. None of the above

31. Chromosome theory of heredity was proposed by

a. Weissmann
b. W.S.Sutton
c. J.G.Mendel
d. None of the above

32. The stain used for G banding is

a. Giemsa
b. Garnet red
c. Glutamin
d. None of the above

33. Which of the following conditions is not specific for a population in Hardy Weinberg equilibrium

a. Random mating
b. Large
c. Absence of migration
d. Geographic isolation

34. Inter-allelic interaction of genes is

a. Dominance
b. Epistasis
c. Overdominance
d. All the above

35. If the cetromere of the chromosome is at one end it is known as

a. Telocentric
b. Metacentric
c. Acrocentric
d. Submetacentric

36. Which of the following mechanism doesn't affect genetic recombination in bacteria

a. Transduction
b. Transformation
c. Conjugation
d. Translation

37. Name the organelle in the cell with extranuclear DNA

a. Lysosomes
b. Mitochondria
c. Both a and b
d. None of the above

38. Sex influenced genes are located on

a. X chromosome
b. Y chromosome
c. X and Y chromosome
d. Autosomes

39. Crossing over percentage between two genes will not exceed

a. 25 b. 50

c. 37.5 d. 100

40. Intra-locus interaction of genes is

a. Dominance b. Epistasis

c. Overdominance d. All of the above

41. The genes that change the phenotypic effects of other genes in a quantitative fashion are called

a. Modifiers b. Interfering genes

c. Dominant genes d. None of the above

42. The percentage of individuals in which a character is expressed is

a. Expressivity b. Penetrance

c. Both a and b d. None of the above

43. If the cetromere of the chromosome is at the middle, the chromosome is known as

a. Telocentric b. Metacentric

c. Acrocentric d. Submetacentric

44. Which of the following is an example of sex linked condition

a. Barred condition in poultry

b. Mahogony colour in Ayshire cattle

c. Baldness in man

d. Horned condition in sheep

45. The occurrence of mutation without any specific cause is called

a. Induced mutation b. Point mutation

c. Spontaneous mutation d. None of the above

46. Heterogametic females are seen in

a. Cattle b. Poultry

c. Honey bee d. Drosophila

47. Barrbody is inactivated

a. Y chromosome b. X chromosome

c. Sex chromosome d. Autosome

48. Heritability estimate in an inbred population will be

a) High b) Zero
c) Low d) One

49. Appearance of ancestral trait after some generations is

a) Mutation b) Reappearance
c) Atavism d) None of the above

50. Traits controlled by genes in sex chromosomes

a) Sex linked b) Sex influenced
c) Sex limited d) None of the above

51. The DNA is a double helix and its two strands are

a) Parallel b) Independent
c) Anti-parallel d) Co-linear

52. If the recombination frequency is between zero and 0.5, then it is

a) In complete linkage b) Complete linkage
c) No linkage d) Noneof the above

53. Which of the following systematic processes is/are involved in change of gene frequencies

a) Selection b) Mutation
c) Migration d) All of the above

54. In calculation of heritability in broad sense, which is not part of numerator

a) V_A b) V_D
c) V_I d) V_E

55. In Bosindicus the Y chromosomes are

a) Submetacentric b) Acrocentric
c) Metacentric d) Telocentric

56. The concept of dosage compensation is put forward by

a) Lyon b) Bridges
c) Mendel d) Barr

57. In recessive epistasis, the F_2 phenotypic ratio will be

a) 9:3:3:1 b) 12:3:1
c) 13:3 d) 9:3:4

58. In dominant-recessive epistasis, the F_2 phenotypic ratio will be

a) 9:3:4 b) 12:3:1
c) 13:3 d) 9:3:3:1

59. In Eukaryotic cells, the protein synthesis occurs in

a) Mitochondria b) Golgi apparatus
c) Ribosomes d) None of the above

60. The differentiation of spermatids to form sperm is called as

a) Sperm formation b) Spermatogenesis
c) Spermiogenesis d) Spermatolysis

61. The process of exchange of genetic material between two living bacteria by direct contact is called

a) Transformation b) Transduction
c) Conjugation d) Sexduction

62. The resting stage of cell cycle is also known as

a) Interphase b) Prophase
c) Anaphase d) Resting phase

63. During cytokinesis stage of cell division, what will happen to the cell

a) Pairing of chromosomes b) Division of cytoplasm
c) Synthesis of DNA d) Separation of centrioles

64. Changes in chromosome number due to addition or deletion of whole sets of chromosomes is called

a) Duplication b) Aneuploidy
c) Euploidy d) Translocation

65. The chromosome nomenclature 47, +21 in human indicates

a) Klinefelter's syndrome b) Patau syndrome
c) Down syndrome d) Double X syndrome

66. The proportionate reduction in the gametic contribution of particular genotype when compared with a standard genotype is called

a) Coefficient of selection
b) Selective value
c) Selection response
d) Breeding value

67. The value of an individual judged by the mean value of its progeny is called

a) Phenotypic value
b) Genotypic value
c) Average effect
d) Breeding value

68. Which factor given below is not a component of producing ability

a) Additive genetic variance
b) Non-additive genetic variance
c) Permanent environmental effect
d) Temporary environmental effect

69. Given below are the factors influencing gene frequency of a population. Find out the odd one.

a) Selection
b) Genetic drift
c) Mutation
d) Migration

70. In eukaryotes the synthesis of messenger RNA is catalyzed by

a) RNA Polymerase I
b) RNA polymerase II
c) DNA ligase
d) None of the above

71. A condition in which only one allele is sufficient for expression of a trait is known as

a) Homozygous
b) Hemizygous
c) Heterozygous
d) Unizygous

72. Synthesis of RNA from DNA is termed as

a) Transformation
b) Transduction
c) Translation
d) Transcription

73. The contribution of offspring to the next generation is known as

a) Selection coefficient
b) Fitness
c) Response
d) Genetic load

74. The frequency of carriers in a population can be estimated by the formula

a) 2q (1-p) b) pq
c) 2p (1-p) d) pq (1-p)

75. Heritability ranges between

a) 0 and 1 b) - 8 and + 8
c) - 1and +1 d) 0 and + 8

76. The frequencies of genotypes in a particular locus must be add up to

a) One or unity
b) 50 % of gene frequencies
c) 10 to 50% of gene frequencies
d) 10 %of gene frequencies

77. Heritability estimates can be increased by

a) Reducing the V_A b) Increasing the V_E
c) Increasing the V_A d) Both a and b

78. Creeper condition in domestic fowl is due to

a) Epistasis b) Co-dominance
c) Semi dominant lethal gene d) None of the above

79. Particulate and duplicate nature of hereditary factors or elements was first demonstrated by

a) William Bateson b) R.C. Punnett
c) G.J. Mendel d) C.F. Wolff

80. If there are more than two alleles at a locus in a population, they are called

a) Multiple alleles b) Isoalleles
c) Pseudo alleles d) None of the above

81. If two genes are copies of an ancestral gene then they are called

a) Alike in state b) Identical by descent
c) Homozygous d) None of the above

82. One of the important evolutionary force is

a) Gene frequency
b) Genetic equilibrium
c) Random drift
d) None of the above

83. Systematic processes operate in

a) Large population
b) Small population
c) Medium population
d) Both a and b

84. In case of HW equilibrium, the frequency of q can be calculated by the formula

a) u/ u+v
b) S_1 / (S_1+S_2)
c) v/ u+v
d) None of the above

85. The phenomena in which the crossing over at one point decreases the probability of occurrence elsewhere on the same chromosome is called

a) Double crossing over
b) Interference
c) Chiasma
d) Coincidence

86. The diploid chromosome number in dogs is

a) 60
b) 50
c) 78
d) 58

87. Multiple allele occupy the

a) Same loci and affect same trait
b) Different loci and affect same trait
c) Same loci and affect different trait
d) Different loci and different trait

88. In an equilibrium population, if gene frequencies of two alleles among the parents are p and q, then the genotype frequency of heterozygotes is

a) p^2
b) q^2
c) pq
d) 2pq

89. In a metaphase stage the chromosomes are

a) Condensed
b) Lengthy
c) Seen with bands
d) Distributed in the cell

90. Parthenogenesis means

a) Unfertilized eggs developing into new individual
b) Tendency to revert to ancestral type
c) Fertility between two species
d) Reproduction through union of male and female gametes

91. Assuming a population in Hardy-Weinberg equilibrium, if the gene frequency of a recessive allele is 0.4, then the genotypic frequency of heterozygotes is

a) 0.48 b) 0.20
c) 0.24 d) 0.16

92. If the mean environmental deviation in a population is zero, then the mean phenotypic value is equal to the mean

a) Genotypic value b) Phenotypic value
c) Dominance deviation d) Interaction deviation

93. The magnitude of genetic drift is larger when the population size is

a) Large b) Small
c) Medium d) Idealized population

94. Number of generations required to change the gene frequency from q_o to q_t is

a) $t = (1/q_o - 1/q_t)$ b) $t = (1/q_t - 1/q_o)$
c) $t = (1/q_o$ d) None of the above

95. The chromosome complement of a ewe is

a) 54, XX b) 54, XY
c) 60, XX d) 52, XY

96. Histones are proteins rich in lysine and arginine and are

a) Neutral b) Negatively charged
c) Positively charged d) None of the above

97. DNA replication always takes place in

a) 5′ to 3′ direction b) 3′ to 5′ direction
c) 3′ to 3′ direction d) None of the above

98. Sense codon among the following is

a) UGA b) UAC

c) UAA d) UAG

99. Anticodons are present in

a) t RNA b) m RNA

c) hn RNA d) r RNA

100. A chromosome with arms of equal length is termed as

a) Sub metacentric b) Metacentric

c) Telocentric d) Acrocentric

101. Sudden heritable change in the structure of gene is

a) Atavism b) Mutation

c) Meiosis d) Random drift

102. In a typical dihybrid cross, the proportion of F_2 genotypes that are heterozygous for both the gene pairs is

a) 1/16 b) 2/16

c) 4/16 d) 8/16

103. Which of the following properties is false with respect to the genetic code

a) Universal b) Triplet code

c) Overlapping d) Degenerate

104. If adenine makes up 15% if bases in a DNA sample, cytosine bases must be

a) 15% b) 35%

c) 30% d) 85%

105. Which of the following is (are) due to semi dominant lethal condition

a) Creeper fowl b) Yellow coat color in mice

c) Both a and b d) None of the above

106. Thymine dimers in the DNA are caused by

a) UV rays b) Transposons

c) Base analogs d) Acridine dyes

107. The dispersive process operates mostly in

a) Large population
b) Small population
c) Both a and b
d) None of the above

108. The chromosomal complement of a Bosindicus bull is

a) 50, XY
b) 64, XY
c) 50, XX
d) 60, XY

109. The preformation theory was proposed by

a) Maupertuis
b) Jan Swammerdam
c) Pythagoras
d) Wolff

110. In dominant epistasis, the F2 phenotypic ratio will be

a) 13:3
b) 12:3:1
c) 9:3:4
d) 9:7

111. Nitrogenous base absent in DNA is

a) Adenine
b) Uracil
c) Guanine
d) Thiamine

112. In test crossing the offspring is crossed with

a) Male parent
b) Female parent
c) Homozygous recessive parent
d) Homozygous dominant parent

113. Appearance of the remote ancestral trait in an individual is termed as

a) Atavism
b) Expressivity
c) Mutation
d) Penetrance

114. A chromosome in which the centromere is exactly at the centre is called

a) Acrocentric
b) Metacentric
c) Sub metacentric
d) Telocentric

115. The following F_2 phenotypic ratio is not an indication of epistatis

a) 1:2:1
b) 9:7
c) 12:3:1
d) 9:6:1

116. Colour blindness and haemophilia in human beings are examples for

a) Sex linked traits b) Sex limited traits
c) Co-dominant inheritance d) Sex influenced traits

117. Which of the following is not a component of repeatability or producing ability

a) Non additive genetic variance
b) Additive genetic variance
c) Temporary environmental variance
d) Permanent environmental variance

118. Heritability estimate ranges between

a) - 1 to +1 b) 0 to 1
c) 0 to + á d) -á to + á

119. The Mendel's law of random assortment is based on

a) Mono hybrid cross b) Dihybrid cross
c) Back cross d) Test cross

120. The sudden heritable change in the genetic material is called

a) Mutation b) Penetrance
c) Atavism d) Expressivity

121. The genes that change the phenotypic effects of other genes in a quantitative fashion are known as

a) Modifiers b) Killers
c) Jumping genes d) Segregators

122. The intra allelic interaction is otherwise known as

a) Epistasis b) Dominance
c) Both a and B d) None of the above

123. RNA differs from DNA by containing

a) Deoxyribose sugar b) Ribose sugar
c) Nitrogen base d) None of the above

124. ZZ-ZW system of sex determination is seen in

a) Drosophila b) Grasshopper
c) Birds d) Human

125. 6) Name the organelle in the cell with extranuclear DNA

a) Ribosome b) Mitochondria
c) Golgi body d) None of the above

126. Chromosomes normally occur as homologous pairs in

a) Zygote b) Egg cell
c) Sperm cell d) Gamete

127. MN blood group system is an example of

a. Dominance b. Partial dominance
c. Co dominance d. Over dominance

128. Barr body is inactivated

a. Y chromosome b. X chromosome
c. Sex chromosome d. Autosome

129. The mutation in which a purine is replaced by another purine is termed as

a. Transversion b Transduction
c. Transition d. None of the above

130. The process to increase the frequency of desirable genes without creating or introducing new one is known as

a) Crossbreeding b) Inbreeding
c) Selection d) None of the above

131. The genetic correlation between milk yield and fat percentage is

a) Positive b) Negative
c) Zero d) One

132. The phenotype is a good indicator of the genotype when the heritability of a character is

a) High b) Medium
c) Low d) None of the above

133. The correlation between repeated measurements in the same animal is defined as

a) Correlation b) Repeatability
c) Combining ability d) Heritability

134. Selection is efficient tool for genetic improvement in farm animals because it,

a) Creates new genes
b) Increases frequency of desirable genes
c) Provides favorable environment
d) None of these

135. Movement of breeding animals into a population is termed as

a) Immigration b) Emigration
c) Mutation d) Genetic drift

136. One of the important evolutionary forces is

a) Gene frequency b) Genetic equilibrium
c) Random drift d) None of the above

137. A mutational event that recurs with characteristic frequency is

a) Reverse mutation b) Non-recurrent mutation
c) Recurrent mutation d) Constant mutation

138. Mutations that do not bring about visible changes in the phenotype are called

a) Gross mutation b) Silent mutation
c) Non-sense mutation d) Zero mutation

139. The effect of migration in a population can be predicted

a) Both in amount and direction
b) In amount only
c) In direction only
d) None of the above

140. The scientist first to demonstrate Mendelian inheritance of qualitative characters in animals

a) T.H.Morgan b) W.E.Castle
c) William Bateson d) None of the above

141. The particular site or position of a gene in a chromosome is known as

a) Genotype
b) Locus
c) Allele
d) Linkage group

142. The structure of DNA was discovered by

a) Watson and Crick
b) Friedrich Miescher
c) Rosalind Franklin
d) None of the above

143. The main function of mitochondria is

a) Synthesis of proteins
b) Synthesis of enzymes
c) Oxidation and release of energy
d) None of the above

144. If the phenotypic value of the heterozygote exceeds the value of both homozygotes, then it is known as

a) Dominance
b) Overdominance
c) Incomplete dominance
d) None of the above

145. In ABO blood group system with three alleles (I^A I^B and I^O), if the frequency of I^A and I^B in a population were 0.20 and 0.40 respectively,then frequency of I^O will be

a) 0.4
b) 0.3
c) 0.7
d) 1.0

146. The assemblage of genes possessed by an individual in pairs is called

a) Gene frequency
b) Gene substitution
c) Gene combination
d) Genotype

147. Southern blotting technique is used to study the genetic variation in

a) RNA
b) Protein
c) Chromosome
d) DNA

148. Twins produced from one egg cell and one sperm cell are:

a) Identical
b) Fraternal
c) Maternal
d) None of the above

149. Sickle-cell anaemia, an inherited human disease is due to the substitution of

a) Amino acid
b) Proteins
c) DNA
d) None of the above

150. Crossing over is rare or absent in

a) Female Drosophila
b) Male Drosophila
c) In both
d) None of the above

151. The concept of linkage was given by

a) Thomson
b) G.Johan Mendel
c) Johanson
d) Morgan

152. The "Genic balance theory" was given by

a) Bateson
b) Sturtenant
c) Bridge
d) Waldeyer

153. The concept of genetic map was given by

a) Morgan
b) Sturtenant
c) Darwin
d) Muller

154. The word 'mitosis' was coined by

a) Alexander Fleming
b) Walther Fleming
c) Ian Fleming
d) Ian Gordon

155. The following phenotypic ratio obtained when double heterozygotes are crossed in dominant epistasis.

a) 9 : 7
b) 15 : 1
c) 9: 3: 7
d) 12 : 3 : 1

156. The inheritance of following character is not sex linked

a) Holandric inheritance
b) Colorblindness in man
c) White eye in drosophila
d) Baldness in human being

157. The following is not a structural chromosomal aberration.

a) Inversion
b) Transversion
c) Deletion
d) Translocation

158. The following is not a numerical chromosomal aberration.

a) Turner Syndrome b) Down Syndrome
c) Immune deficiency Syndrome d) Fragile X Syndrome

159. The following statement is true about the components of variance.

a) VA = VI + VD b) VP = VD + VI
c) VG = VA + VD + VI d) VP = VG + VE + VI

160. The following is not a systematic force that changes gene frequency.

a) Population size b) Migration
c) Mutation d) Selection

KEY

1. a) One
2. c) Mutation
3. b) Heterogametic
4. c) Isochromosomes
5. b) Metaphase
6. b) 54,XY
7. b) Spallanzani
8. c) Man with blood group AB
9. c) 64
10. d) 9:3:3:1
11. c) Holandric inheritance
12. c) Migration
13. d) 47
14. c) 1:2:1
15. a) Co-dominant
16. a) Distance between them
17. d) 24
18. c) Back cross
19. b) Colchicine
20. a) Sex linked traits
21. a) Sons only
22. c) Both males and females
23. a) Weissmann
24. a) Positive
25. b) Males
26. d) Rose x Pea
27. b) Law of purity of gametes
28. b) Female
29. a) Dominant & recessive epistasis
30. a) W. Johanssen
31. b) W.S.Sutton
32. a) Giemsa
33. d) Geographic isolation
34. b) Epistasis
35. a) Telocentric
36. a) Translation
37. b) Mitochondria
38. d) Autosomes
39. b) 50%
40. a) Dominance
41. a) Modifiers

42. b) Penetrance
43. b) Metacentric
44. a) Barred condition in poultry
45. c) Spontaneous mutation
46. b) Poultry
47. b) X chromosome
48. c) Low
49. c) Atavism
50. a) Sex linked
51. c) Anti-parallel
52. a) Incomplete linkage
53. d) All the above
54. d) V_E
55. b) Acrocentric
56. a) Lyon
57. d) 9:3:4
58. c) 13:3
59. c) Ribosomes
60. c) Spermiogenesis
61. c) Conjugation
62. a) Interphase
63. b) Division of cytoplasm
64. c) Euploidy
65. c) Down syndrome
66. a) Coefficient of selection
67. d) Breeding value
68. d) Temporary environmental effect
69. b) Genetic drift
70. b) RNA polymerase II
71. b) Hemizygous
72. d) Transcription
73. b) Fitness
74. c) 2p (1-p)
75. a) 0 and 1
76. a) One or unity
77. c) Increasing the V_A
78. c) Semi dominant lethal gene
79. c) G.J. Mendel
80. a) Multiple alleles
81. b) Identical by descent
82. c) Random drift
83. a) Large population
84. a) u/ u+v
85. b) Interference
86. c) 78
87. a) Same loci and affect same trait
88. d) 2pq
89. a) Condensed
90. a) Unfertilized eggs developing into new individual
91. a) 0.48
92. a) Genotypic value
93. b) Small
94. b) $t = (1/q_t - 1/q_o)$
95. a) 54, XX
96. c) Positively charged
97. a) 5′ to 3′ direction
98. b) UAC
99. a) t RNA
100. b) Metacentric
101. b) Mutation
102. c) 4/16
103. c) Overlapping
104. b) 35%

105. a) Creeper fowl
106. a) UV rays
107. b) Small population
108. d) 60, XY
109. b) Jan Swammerdam
110. b) 12:3:1
111. b) Uracil
112. c) Homozygous recessive parent
113. a) Atavism
114. b) Metacentric
115. a) 1:2:1
116. a) Sex linked traits
117. c) Temporary environmental variance
118. b) Dihybrid cross
119. a) Mutation
120. c) Homozygous recessive parent
121. a) Modifiers
122. b) Dominance
123. b) Ribose sugar
124. c) Birds
125. b) Mitochondria
126. a) Zygote
127. c) Co dominance
128. b) X chromosome
129. c) Transition
130. c) Selection
131. b) Negative
132. a) High
133. b) Repeatability
134. c) Increases the frequency of desirable genes
135. a) Immigration
136. c) Random drift
137. c) Recurrent mutation
138. b) Silent mutation
139. a) Both in amount and direction
140. c) William Bateson
141. b) Locus
142. a) Watson and Crick
143. c) Oxidation and release of energy
144. b) Over dominance
145. a) 0.4
146. d) Genotype
147. d) DNA
148. a) Identical
149. a) Amino acid
150. b) Male Drosophila
151. c) Johanson
152. c) Bridge
153. b) Sturtenant
154. b) Walther Fleming
155. d) 12:3:1
156. d) Baldness in human being
157. b) Transversion
158. c) Immune Deficiuency Syndrome
159. c) VG= VA + VD + VI
160. a) Population Size

4. Match the Following

SET I

1.	Point mutation	a.	47, +13
2.	Alkylating agents	b.	Additive value
3.	Mitogen	c.	38
4.	XX-XY sex determination	d.	b_{AP}
5.	XX-XO sex determination	e.	78
6.	Turner's syndrome	f.	Nitrogen mustard
7.	Patau syndrome	g.	Change in single base pair
8.	Breeding value	h.	45, XO
9.	Chromosome number of pigs	i.	Bateson
10.	Chromosome number of sheep	j.	J.L. Lush
11.	Chromosome number of chicken	k.	C.B. Bridges
12.	Repeatability	l.	54
13.	Heritability	m.	Drosophila
14.	Genetics	n.	Phytohameagglutinin
15.	Balance concept	o.	Grass hopper

SET II

1.	Heritability in broad sense	a.	Additive genetic variance
2.	Genetic correlation	b.	0 to 8
3.	Major genes	c.	Random mating
4.	Growth traits	d.	Pleiotropy
5.	Gene frequency	e.	Qualitative characters
6.	Heritability in narrow sense	f.	High heritability
7.	Panmixia	g.	V_G/V_P
8.	Breeding value	h.	0 to 1
9.	Reproductive traits	i.	Quantitative characters
10.	Minor genes	j.	Quantitative characters
		k.	V_G/V_P

SET III

1.	Plastid	a.	Holandric
2.	13:3	b.	Synthesis of m – RNA
3.	3n	c.	Genic Balance Theory
4.	Webbed toes	d.	Similar genes
5.	Hb_S	e.	Dominant epistasis
6.	Homozygous	f.	Gene
7.	Transcription	g.	Euploidy
8.	C.B. Bridges	h.	Dominant & recessive epistasis
9.	Johanssen	i.	Sickle cell anemia
10.	12:3:1	j.	Extra chromosomal inheritance

SET IV

1. Small population	a. b_{AP}
2. Non-genetic factors	b. Carrier
3. Quantitative trait	c. Proportion of particular genotype
4. Qualitative traits	d. Environment
5. Heritability	e. 1- Selection coefficient
6. Genotype frequency	f. Migration
7. Heterozygote	g. Random drift
8. Movement of animals	h. ¼ V_E/V_P
	i. Continuous variation
	j. Influenced by one or few genes

SET V

1. Bull dog appearance	a. Sex linked lethal
2. Paramecium	b. 13:3
3. Duplicate dominant epistasis	c. Sickle cell anaemia
4. Inheritance of acquired characters	d. 9:7
5. Haemophilia	e. Cytoplasmic inheritance
6. Start codon	f. Lamark
7. Pangenesis	g. AUG
8. Duplicate recessive epistasis	h. Charles Darwin
9. Mutation	i. 15:1
10. Recessive and dominant epistasis	j. Semi-dominant lethal
	k. 9:3:4

SET VI

1. Polytene chromosome	a. 'n' number of chromosomes
2. 1/29 chromosomes	b. Quantitative inheritance
3. Co-dominance	c. Down's syndrome
4. Linkage and crossing over	d. Morgan
5. Sex linked inheritance	e. Robertsonian translocation
6. Trisomy	f. Dipteria
7. Incomplete dominance	g. ABO blood group
8. Kernal color in wheat	h. White eye in drosophila
9. Selection	i. Blue color in poultry
10. Spermatozoa	j. Differential rate of reproduction

SET VII

1. Multiple alleles	a. Small population
2. Epistasis	b. Linkage
3. Spermatid	c. Sex linked characters
4. Genetic correlation	d. 1:1
5. Genetic drift	e. Blood groups
6. Test cross ratio	f. Sex mosaic
7. Skip gap inheritance	g. Haploid chromosome
8. Gynandromorph	h. 15:1

SET VIII

1. Barr body	a. Holandric
2. Rabbit coat color	b. Monosomy
3. 47 chromosomes	c. Genic balance theory
4. Y chromosome	d. Dihybrid test cross ratio
5. Pyrimidine	e. Recessive epistasis
6. 1:1:1:1	f. Germplasm theory
7. 2n-1	g. Down's syndrome
8. C.B.Bridges	h. Multiple alleles
9. Weismann	i. Cytosine
10. 9:3:4	j. Sec chromatin

SET IX

1. Dominant and recessive epistasis	a. 12:3:1
2. Plumage in Andulasian chicken	b. Nitrogen mustard
3. Comb pattern in poultry	c. Codominance
4. Coat color in rabbits	d. 13:3
5. Achondroplasia in cattle	e. Cytoplasmic inheritance
6. Alkylating agents	f. Multiple alleles
7. Coat color in short horn cattle of genes	g. Complementary interaction
8. Dominant epistasis	h. $(V_G+V_{EP}) / V_P$
9. Genetic correlations	i. $h_X.h_Y.r_A$
10. Shell coiling in snails	j. Incomplete penetrance
11. Repeatability	k. Semi dominant lethals
12. Co-heritability	l. Pleiotropy

SET X

1.	Arthur Kornberg	a.	Sex chromatin
2.	Watson and Crick	b.	Base composition of DNA
3.	Beadle and Tatum	c.	First artificial synthesis of DNA
4.	Landsteiner	d.	DNA as hereditary material
5.	Morgan	e.	Variance ratio test
6.	H.G. Khorana	f.	One gene One enzyme hypothesis
7.	Avery, McLeod and McCarty	g.	Double helical structure of DNA
8.	Murray Barr	h.	ABO blood groups in human
9.	Fisher	i.	DNA polymerase
10.	Chargaff	j.	Linkage and crossing over

SET XI

1.	Monosomy	a.	Carries n number of chromosomes
2.	1/29 chromosomes	b.	Discontinuous variation
3.	Multiple alleles	c.	Down's syndrome
4.	Rose X pea comb	d.	Robertsonian translocation
5.	Crossing over	e.	Gene interaction
6.	Trisomy	f.	2n-1
7.	Incomplete dominance	g.	ABO blood groups
8.	Kernalcolour in wheat	h.	Copy choice
9.	Quantitative trait	i.	Blue color in poultry
10.	Spermatozoa	j.	Baldness
11.	Theory of evolution	k.	Walnut
12.	Lethal gene	l.	Yellow color in mice
13.	Sex influenced trait	m.	2n= 60
14.	Qualitative trait	n.	Charles Darwin
15.	Goat	o.	Polygenes

SET XII

1.	Heritability in narrow sense	a.	Pleiotropy
2.	Inbreeding	b.	Morgan
3.	Origin of species	c.	J.L.Lush
4.	Genetic correlation	d.	Equal chance of mating
5.	Panmixia	e.	Small population
6.	Baldness	f.	V_A/V_P
7.	Heritability in broad sense	g.	Sex linked trait
8.	Egg production in poultry	h.	V_G/V_P
9.	Repeatability	i.	Charles Darwin
10.	Linkage and crossing over	j.	Sex limited trait
		k.	Sex influenced trait

SET XIII

1.	Non genetic factors	a.	Copy choice
2.	Genetic correlation	b.	Nitrogen Mustard
3.	Reproductive traits	c.	Discrete variation
4.	MPPA	d.	Environment
5.	Crossing over	e.	Cytosine
6.	Pyrimidine	f.	Spermatozoa
7.	Alkylating agent	g.	Continuous variation
8.	Quantitative traits	h.	Pleiotrophy
9.	Qualitative traits	i.	Low heritability
10.	Haploid set of chromosome	j.	ABO blood groups
		k.	Repeatability

SET XIV

1.	Dog	a) human female
2.	Morgan	b) additive effect of genes
3.	Muller	c) XO
4.	Eye colour Drosophila	d) 2N= 78
5.	Law of purity of gamete	e) Plasma gene
6.	Pig	f) sex linked
7.	Erethroblastosisfetalis	g) linkage
8.	Breeding value	h) X ray mutation genes
9.	Cytoplasmic inheritance	i) 2N= 38
10.	Turner's Syndrome	j) Segregation

KEY

SET I

1.	Point mutation	g.	Change in single base pair
2.	Alkylating agents	f.	Nitrogen mustard
3.	Mitogen	n.	Phytohameagglutinin
4.	XX-XY sex determination	m.	Drosophila
5.	XX-XO sex determination	o.	Grass hopper
6.	Turner's syndrome	h.	45, XO
7.	Patau syndrome	a.	47, +13
8.	Breeding value	d.	b_{AP}
9.	Chromosome number of pigs	c.	38
10.	Chromosome number of sheep	l.	54
11.	Chromosome number of chicken	e.	78
12.	Repeatability	j.	J.L. Lush
13.	Heritability	b.	Additive value
14.	Genetics	i.	Bateson
15.	Balance concept	k.	C.B. Bridges

SET II

1.	Heritability in broad sense	g.	V_G/V_P
2.	Genetic correlation	d.	Pleiotropy
3.	Major genes	e.	Qualitative characters
4.	Growth traits	f.	High heritability
5.	Gene frequency	h.	0 to 1
6.	Heritability in narrow sense	k.	V_A/V_P
7.	Panmixia	c.	Random mating
8.	Breeding value	a.	Additive genetic variance
9.	Reproductive traits	j.	Low heritability
10.	Minor genes	i.	Quantitative characters

SET III

1.	Plastid	j.	Extra chromosomal inheritance
2.	13:3	h.	Dominant & recessive epistasis
3.	3n	g.	Euploidy
4.	Webbed toes	a.	Holandric
5.	HbS	i.	Sickle cell anemia
6.	Homozygous	d.	Similar genes
7.	Transcription	b.	Synthesis of m—RNA
8.	C.B. Bridges	c.	Genic Balance Theory
9.	Johanssen	f.	Gene
10.	12:3:1	e.	Dominant epistasis

SET IV

1.	Small population	g.	Random drift
2.	Non-genetic factors	d.	Environment
3.	Quantitative trait	i.	Continuous variation
4.	Qualitative traits	j.	Influenced by one or few genes
5.	Heritability	a.	b_{AP}
6.	Genotype frequency	c.	Proportion of particular genotype
7.	Heterozygote	b.	Carrier
8.	Movement of animals	f.	Migration

SET V

1.	Bull dog appearance	j.	Semi-dominant lethal
2.	Paramecium	e.	Cytoplasmic inheritance
3.	Duplicate dominant epistasis	i.	15:1
4.	Inheritance of acquired characters	f.	Lamark

5.	Haemophilia	a.	Sex linked lethal
6.	Start codon	g.	AUG
7.	Pangenesis	h.	Charles Darwin
8.	Duplicate recessive epistasis	d.	9:7
9.	Mutation	c.	Sickle cell anaemia
10.	Recessive and dominant epistasis	b.	13:3

SET VI

1.	Polytene chromosome	f.	Dipteria
2.	1/29 chromosomes	e.	Robertsonian translocation
3.	Co-dominance	g.	ABO blood group
4.	Linkage and crossing over	d.	Morgan
5.	Sex linked inheritance	h.	White eye in drosophila
6.	Trisomy	c.	Down's syndrome
7.	Incomplete dominance	i.	Blue color in poultry
8.	Kernal color in wheat	b.	Quantitative inheritance
9.	Selection	j.	Differential rate of reproduction
10.	Spermatozoa	a.	'n' number of chromosomes

SET VII

1.	Multiple alleles	e.	Blood groups
2.	Epistasis	h.	15:1
3.	Spermatid	g.	Haploid chromosome
4.	Genetic correlation	b.	Linkage
5.	Genetic drift	a.	Small population
6.	Test cross ratio	d.	1:1
7.	Skip gap inheritance	c.	Sex linked characters
8.	Gynandromorph	f.	Sex mosaic

SET VIII

1.	Barr body	j.	Sex chromatin
2.	Rabbit coat color	h.	Multiple alleles
3.	47 chromosomes	g.	Down's syndrome
4.	Y chromosome	a.	Holandric
5.	Pyrimidine	i.	Cytosine
6.	1:1:1:1	d.	Dihybrid test cross ratio
7.	2n-1	b.	Monosomy
8.	C.B.Bridges	c.	Genic balance theory
9.	Weismann	f.	Germplasm theory
10.	9:3:4	e.	Recessive epistasis

SET IX

1.	Dominant and recessive epistasis	d.	13:3
2.	Plumage in Andulasian chicken	j.	Incomplete penetrance
3.	Comb pattern in poultry	g.	Complementary interaction of genes
4.	Coat color in rabbits	f.	Multiple alleles
5.	Achondroplasia in cattle	k.	Semi dominant lethal
6.	Alkylating agents	b.	Nitrogen mustard
7.	Coat color in short horn cattle	c.	Co-dominance
8.	Dominant epistasis	a.	12:3:1
9.	Genetic correlations	l.	Pleiotropy
10.	Shell coiling in snails	e.	Cytoplasmic inheritance
11.	Repeatability	h.	$(V_G+V_{EP}) / V_P$
12.	Co-heritability	i.	$h_X.h_Y.r_A$

SET X

1.	Arthur Kornberg	i.	DNA polymerase
2.	Watson and Crick	g.	Double helical structure of DNA
3.	Beadle and Tatum	f.	One gene One enzyme hypothesis
4.	Landsteiner	h.	ABO blood groups in human
5.	Morgan	j.	Linkage and crossing over
6.	H.G. Khorana	c.	First artificial synthesis of DNA
7.	Avery, McLeod and McCarty	d.	DNA as hereditary material
8.	Murray Barr	a.	Sex chromatin
9.	Fisher	e.	Variance ratio test
10.	Chargaff	b.	Base composition of DNA

SET XI

1.	Monosomy	f.	2n-1
2.	1/29 chromosomes	d.	Robertsonian translocation
3.	Multiple alleles	g.	ABO blood groups
4.	Rose X pea comb	k.	Walnut
5.	Crossing over	h.	Copy choice
6.	Trisomy	c.	Down's syndrome
7.	Incomplete dominance	i.	Blue color in poultry
	Kernalcolour in wheat	e.	Gene interaction
8.	Quantitative trait	o.	Polygenes
9.	Spermatozoa	a.	Carries n number of chromosomes

10. Theory of evolution	n. Charles Darwin
11. Lethal gene	l. Yellow color in mice
12. Sex influenced trait	j. Baldness
13. Qualitative trait	b. Discontinuous variation
14. Goat	m. 2n= 60

SET XII

1. Heritability in narrow sense	f. V_A/V_P
2. Inbreeding	e. Small population
3. Origin of species	i. Charles Darwin
4. Genetic correlation	a. Pleiotropy
5. Panmixia	d. Equal chance of mating
6. Baldness	k. Sex influenced trait
7. Heritability in broad sense	h. V_G/V_P
8. Egg production in poultry	j. Sex limited trait
9. Repeatability	c. J.L.Lush
10. Linkage and crossing over	b. Morgan

SET XIII

1. Non genetic factors	d. Environment
2. Genetic correlation	h. Pleiotrophy
3. Reproductive traits	i. Low heritability
4. MPPA	k. Repeatability
5. Crossing over	a. Copy choice
6. Pyrimidine	e. Cytosine
7. Alkylating agent	b. Nitrogen Mustard
8. Quantitative traits	g. Continuous variation
9. Qualitative traits	c. Discrete variation
10. Haploid set of chromosome	f. Spermatozoa

SET XIV

1. Dog	d. 2N= 78
2. Morgan	g. linkage
3. Muller	h. X ray mutation genes
4. Eye colour Drosophila	f. sex linked d)
5. Law of purity of gamete	j. Segregation
6. Pig	i. 2N= 38
7. Erethroblastosisfetalis	a. human female g)
8. Breeding value	b. additive effect of genes
9. Cytoplasmic inheritance	e. Plasma gene
10. Turner's Syndrome	c. XO

5. Define the Following

1. Allele
2. Atavism
3. Average effect
4. Back cross
5. Degeneracy
6. Breeding value
7. Carrier
8. Co-dominance
9. Coefficient of fitness
10. Continuous variation
11. Correlation
12. Criss-cross inheritance
13. Crossing over
14. Discontinuous variation
15. Dispersive process
16. DNA
17. Dominance
18. Effective population size
19. Environment
20. Point mutation
21. Epistasis
22. Expressivity
23. Fitness
24. Polymorphism
25. Gene frequency
26. Generation interval
27. Genetic code
28. Genetics
29. Genotype
30. Polysomes
31. Plasmids
32. Genotype frequency
33. Hardy-Weinberg law
34. Heredity
35. Heritability in broad sense
36. Nonsense codons
37. Heritability in narrow sense
38. Incomplete dominance
39. Karyotype
40. Law of random assortment
41. Law of segregation
42. Lethal genes
43. Linkage
44. Load
45. Locus
46. Meiosis
47. Multiple alleles
48. Mutation
49. Oogenesis
50. Over dominance
51. Panmixia
52. Penetrance
53. Phenocopy
54. Phenotype
55. Pleiotropy
56. Population
57. Population mean
58. Prepotency
59. Protein synthesis
60. Purine
61. Pyrimidine
62. Qualitative traits
63. Quantitative traits
64. Repeatability

65. RNA
66. Sex influenced traits
67. Sex limited traits
68. Sex linked traits
69. Spermatogenesis
70. Systematic process
71. Test cross
72. Value
73. Transposons
74. Totipotent

6. Differentiate Between the Following

1. Additive and non-additive gene action
2. Coefficient of selection and fitness
3. Coupling and repulsion relationship
4. Dominance and over dominance
5. Incomplete dominance and partial dominance
6. Fertility and viability
7. Somatic and germinal mutations
8. Fitness and coefficient of selection
9. DNA and RNA
10. Epistasis and dominance
11. Forward and reverse mutations
12. Natural and artificial selection
13. Gene and genotype frequencies
14. General and special environment
15. Half sibs and full sibs
16. Interference and co-incidence coefficient
17. Linkage and crossing over
18. Mitosis and Meiosis
19. Monohybrid and dihybrid cross
20. Multiple allele and multiple factor
21. Penetrance and expressivity of gene
22. Additive and non-additive gene action
23. Population genetics and quantitative genetics

24. Prokaryotes and Eukaryotes
25. Purine and pyrimidine
26. Quantitative and qualitative traits
27. Random and non-random mating
28. Sex linked and sex limited inheritance
29. Systematic and dispersive process
30. Transcription and translation
31. Genetic and phenotypic correlations
32. Spermatogenesis and oogenesis
33. Translocation and crossing over
34. Preformation theory and vapour theory
35. Heritability in narrow and broad sense

7. Write Short Notes on the Following

1. Among autosomal and sex linked recessive lethal, which one is easy to identify? Explain
2. Aneuploidy
3. Atavism
4. Auto-sexing in poultry
5. Blending inheritance
6. Genetic markers
7. Breeding under unfavourable climate
8. Breeding value
9. Classification of chromosomal aberrations
10. Classification of various modifications of dihybrid ratio
11. ClB technique
12. Co-dominance
13. Coefficient of inbreeding
14. Components of phenotypic variance

15. Coupling and repulsion phase of linkage
16. Crossing over
17. Cytoplasmic inheritance
18. Deficiency
19. Developmental genetics
20. Do you think that somatic cell mutation will be transmitted to the progeny in domestic animals? Explain
21. Dominance deviation
22. Duplicate dominant epistasis
23. Effect of mutation on gene frequency
24. Epistasis
25. Extrachromosal inheritance
26. Forces that cause change in gene and genotype frequencies
27. Genetic constitution of the population in terms of gene and genotype frequencies
28. Genic balance theory of sex determination
29. Grading up
30. Heritability
31. Inheritance of blood group in human being
32. Inheritance of coat color in rabbit
33. Is it a good policy to breed Dexters to Dexters to produce Dexter offspring? Explain
34. Kappa particles
35. Law of segregation with example
36. Lethal genes
37. Linkage
38. Mapping of chromosomes
39. Mendel's law of independent assortment
40. Milk factor in mice
41. Modifiers

42. Mosaic dominance
43. Most probable producing ability
44. Muller's ClB method
45. Mutagens
46. Mutation
47. Non-disjunction
48. Numerical aberrations of chromosomes
49. Oogenesis
50. Pedigree selection
51. Pleiotropy
52. Polyploidy
53. Population mean
54. Prophase of meiosis
55. Protein synthesis
56. Repeatability and its estimation
57. Effect of selection on gene frequency
58. Sex limited inheritance
59. Sex linked inheritance
60. Significance of meiosis
61. Structural chromosomal aberrations
62. Test cross
63. Theory of pangenesis
64. Uses of Hardy-Weinberg law
65. Various syndromes in man associated with chromosomal aberrations
66. Inheritance of comb pattern in fowl
67. Inheritance of ABO blood group in human being
68. Inheritance of coat color in rodents
69. Watson and Crick model of DNA structure
70. What is the maximum percentage of recombination of genes? Why is it so?

8. Write Essay on the Following

1. Define epistasis. What are the different types of epistasis? Explain any two of them.
2. Describe the various stages of mitosis and meiosis
3. Explain partitioning of phenotypic variance. Write on GE interaction, its impact and ways to reduce it
4. What is meant by systematic process? Explain the effect of various agencies of systematic process on gene frequency
5. What are lethal genes? Classify the various types of lethal gene. How lethal genes can be eliminated from the population?
6. Mention the possible reasons for Mendel's success in conducting his experiment. What is law of segregation and describe it with an example in animals.
7. Describe the chromosomal theory of sex determination in insects, mammals and birds
8. Explain the concept, causes and principal applications of genetic correlation
9. What is mutation? Classify mutations and explain sex linked mutation in brief
10. Write the importance of cytogenetics in livestock. Classify the different chromosomal aberrations
11. State Hardy-Weinberg law. Prove the constancy of gene and genotypic frequencies under Hardy-Weinberg equilibrium
12. Elucidate the structure of DNA as per the works of Watson and Crick. Explain the differences between DNA and RNA
13. Define heritability. Differentiate heritability in broad sense and narrow sense. Write the principle involved in its estimation and write the practical uses of heritability in animal breeding programme
14. Define heritability. Name the different methods of heritability estimation and describe in detail the half sib method of heritability estimation
15. Classify forces influencing gene frequency. How does selection change the gene frequency
16. Define mutagens. Write briefly about chemical mutagens
17. Define linkage and crossing over. Explain linkage as an exception to law of random assortment.

18. Define value and variance. Describe the genetic, phenotypic and environmental variances and their importance in animal breeding
19. Explain the average effect of gene substitution and computation of breeding value based on it.
20. Explain Hardy-Weinberg law giving an example of a biological population with parent generation possessing alleles of A_1 and A_2 in frequencies p and q respectively and $p + q = 1$. What happens when the genetic equilibrium in a population is not disturbed?
21. With the help of autosomal loci explain genetic constitution of a population in terms of genotype and gene frequencies.
22. Define Hardy-Weinberg law. Discuss the conditions required for its application
23. Define mutation. Explain its nature and causes
24. Discuss polygenic inheritance taking milk production in cow as an example
25. Explain interaction of non-allelic genes taking the inheritance of comb shape in poultry as an example
26. Explain sex-linked, sex-influenced and sex limited traits with the help of suitable example in each case.
27. State Mendel's laws of inheritance. Name the seven pairs of contrasting characters studied by Mendel with their dominant and recessive relationship.
28. Explain multiple allelic inheritance of coat colour in rabbits.
29. Classify different categories of gene effect. Discuss additive gene effect.
30. State and explain Mendel's law of segregation and random assortment with suitable examples
31. Differentiate between the quantitative and qualitative traits. Explain multiple factor hypothesis on inheritance of milk yield in dairy cattle
32. Explain the term linkage. Write in detail with suitable example three point crossovers, with double crossover between linked genes are also present.
33. How will you partition the various components of phenotypic variance? Differentiate between narrow and broad sense of heritability
34. Explain the law of independent assortment with special reference to Drosophila's traits

35. Name five sex linked traits and explain their inheritance with special reference to poultry
36. What are the different components of phenotypic variance? Discuss about the various components in detail
37. Define Hardy-Weinberg equilibrium and discuss the various factors affecting the gene frequency
38. Explain the modified Mendelian ratios with examples
39. Define the law of segregation. Discuss in detail the modifications of monohybrid ratio.

□□□

AGB-211 : LIVESTOCK AND POULTRY BREEDING

Section-III

AGB 211 Livestock and Poultry Breeding

1. Fill in the Blanks with Most Suitable Answer

1. ____________________ heritability is estimated from response to selection.
2. Sheep breed reared for pelt is ________________________.
3. __________________ is a native cattle breed of Tamil Nadu known as Jallikattu
4. In pedigree selection more importance should be given to ________________ ancestors.
5. The country where milk recording was first started is ____________________.
6. The deviation in progeny performance from population mean is called ____________________
7. If all individuals in a population are selected the selection differential is ____________________
8. Selection intensity _________________ with increase in variance for the trait.
9. The degree of resemblance between offspring and parent is measured by _________ coefficient.
10. The main force responsible for natural selection is _________________ in a particular environment.

11. The process of removal of poor / inferior animals from the breeding population is called ____________________.

12. __________________ is a term used for individual selection when the selected individuals are all put together for mating.

13. The basis of indirect selection is the high __________________ between the two traits.

14. The environmental effects, which are same for all members of one and the same family are known as ________________________.

15. Karan-Swiss cattle is evolved from Brown Swiss and ____________ breed of cattle.

16. The distinguishing feature of *Bos indicus* is the presence of __________________.

17. The standardized selection differential is also known as ________________.

18. Kangayam is a ____________ purpose breed of cattle in Tamil Nadu.

19. ________________ is the mating of individuals belonging to particular filial generations like F_1 X F_1 or F_2 X F_2

20. The range of Inbreeding coefficient is ____________

21. The breed of cattle produced by crossing Shorthorn, Jersey and local cows around Patna is known as ________________

22. Half sibs have the degree of relationship of __________ while the degree of relationship between grandparent and an individual is __________

23. ________________ is considered as half of the herd

24. Ability of a cow or buffalo to sustain its daily yield for a longer period is termed as ______________________

25. The probability that two genes in a given locus are identical by descent is termed as ________________

26. ________________ is a cross between Male ass (Jack) and female horse (Mare).

27. The agency primarily involved in conservation of animal genetic resources of India is ________________

28. Two basic tools used by animal breeders to make genetic change are __________ and ____________

29. In _____________ mating both parental and maternal heterosis as well as individual heterosis is exploited.
30. The animals having two parents in common are called as ___________
31. Optimum dry period in cattle is_______________
32. In cattle the level of exotic inheritance should be limited to around _______________
33. The milder form of inbreeding is known as _______________
34. The degree of relationship between any two individuals is measured as __________ and named after an American geneticist _____________
35. Reduced fitness of progenies resulting from inbreeding is termed as ___________________
36. Interspecies hybrids do not always propagate because they are generally ________________
37. General combing ability is the property of _______________ while the Specific combining ability is the property of _______________
38. _______________ is the cross between cattle and yak
39. In a breeding pyramid, the topmost tier is _______________
40. In general, selection intensity in male animals will be _______________ where as in female animals it is _______________
41. _______________ is the raw material with which the animal breeder works to bring about genetic improvement through selection.
42. The exotic sheep breed used for developing the crossbred Avivastra is ___________________.
43. _______________ is an important tool to change the gene frequencies in desired direction.
44. The heterozygosity is increased in ___________________ breeding method.
45. Calving interval is the sum of service period and _______________.
46. Unmasking of the lethal recessive genes occurs in _______________ cross
47. The mating system that should be followed in seed stock herds but not in commercial herds is ___________________.

48. Crossing of the inbred lines derived from different breeds is known as ____________________.

49. The ________________ gene action is not responsible for heterosis.

50. Mating of the individuals which are less closely related to each other than the average relationship of the individuals in the population is known as ____________________.

51. Crossing of the F_1 offspring to one of the parent breeds is known as ____________________

52. Current breeding policy to improve the milk production of non-descript buffaloes is ____________________.

53. The system of breeding practiced to retain good proportion of genes of a favoured individual is ____________________.

54. The range of coefficient of inbreeding is ____________________.

55. The minimum number of breeds involved in rotational crossing is ____________________.

56. The ideal calving interval in dairy cattle is ____________________days.

57. The ability of the animal to stamp its characters on its progeny is called ____________________.

58. The method of estimation variance-covariance inbreeding coefficient was given by the Scientist ____________________.

59. The standard lactation length in dairy cattle is ________________ days.

60. Mating of the individuals to improve homozygosity without resorting to inbreeding is known as ____________________ mating.

61. Mating based on phenotype is called ____________________.

62. The coefficient of relationship between half sibs is ________________.

63. Heterosis is due to ________________ gene action.

64. Mating of unrelated purebred individuals within the same breed is called ______________.

65. The genetic effect of out breeding is to increase the proportion of ____________________.

66. When two breeds are crossed alternatively, the method is known as ____________________.

67. In a breeding pyramid, the lower tier is ____________________.

68. The relationship between individuals when one is a descendant of the other is called ____________________.

69. The Buffalo breed with high fat per cent of milk is ____________________

70. ____________________ is a situation wherein heterozygotes usually perform better than the homozygotes.

71. The coefficient of relationship between parent and offspring is ____________________.

72. Two synthetic breeds evolved in India having Brown Swiss inheritance are ____________________ and ____________________.

73. Breeding policy for improving genetic potentiality of Jamnapari goat is ____________________.

74. If inbreeding coefficient of an individual is 0.125 the coefficient of relationship among the parents would be ____________________.

75. Cattalo is the cross between ____________________ and ____________________.

76. Native cattle of India belong to ____________________ species.

77. ____________________ breed of buffalo is largely used for grading up non-descript buffaloes in India.

78. Dividing the selection differential by the phenotypic standard deviation gives ____________________.

79. Selection creates no new ____________________.

80. For a repeatability of 0.60, the accuracy of evaluating an animal on the basis of two records should be increased by ____________________ per cent.

81. Repeatability can be computed as the ____________________ of future performance on past performance.

82. ____________________ is the mating of animals of two or more different breeds while ____________________ is the mating of animals within a breed.

83. Genetic correlation results from ____________________ situation where a gene influences both traits.

84. The system of mating in which relationship of individuals is kept very close to an outstanding ancestor is ____________________.

85. The highest milk yielding cow of the world belongs to ____________________ breed.

86. Best type of selection procedure for carcass traits ________________.

87. Avikalin is a cross between ________________ and ________________.

88. The method of selection in which the correlation between breeding value and calculated value is maximized is called ________________.

89. GMO means ________________________________.

90. A buffalo breed developed by crossing Murrah and Surti is ______________.

91. Selection intensity ________________ with increase in variance for the trait.

92. Estimation of MPPA was introduced by ________________.

93. In animal breeding selection index was introduced by ______________.

94. ______________ method of estimation of heritability is more reliable in cattle

95. The father of taxonomy is ____________________.

96. ________________ is an important tool to change the gene frequencies in desired direction.

97. Henderson (1973) developed a method of sire evaluation which is called as ____________________.

98. When offspring and mid-parent information is used, regression value will be same as ____________ .

99. The precision of an estimate of heritability is indicated by its __________________.

100. The degree of resemblance between offspring and parent is measured by ________ coefficient.

101. In the estimation of repeatability, environmental variance is further partitioned into __________________ and __________________.

102. Repeatability is estimated by __________________________ method.

103. Selection index using information from different sources is known as ______________.

104. The specific combining ability is caused by ________________ genetic effects.

105. In practical breeding, the differential expression of genotypes in different environment is known as __________________.

106. If all the phenotypic variability is genetic in nature, heritability is equal to ______________ .
107. Karan-Swiss cattle is evolved from __________________ and ______________ breeds of cattle.
108. ____________________ method of selection is followed to exploit the non-additive gene action.
109. The amount of selection pressure applied for a particular trait is called as ________________.
110. The practice of improving one trait by selecting on another trait is called ________________.
111. Response to selection is ______________ proportional to the heritability of the trait.
112. ________________ and ______________ were first domesticated species in India.
113. The famous dual purpose breed of cattle of Andhra Pradesh is ________.
114. The basic effect of selection is to change the __________________.
115. To estimate the genetic gain per year of a trait ______________, ______________ and ______________ components are required.
116. ____________ and ___________ are the breed of rabbits which produce white colour fur.
117. The degree of heritability estimate for milk yield in dairy cattle is ________________.
118. The average generation interval for Indian dairy cattle is ___________.
119. ________________ is the first animal to be domesticated.
120. The complications of selection are ____________ and ____________.
121. Genetic constitution of the population is described in terms of __________________ and __________________.
122. __________________ is a group of interbreeding individuals.
123. The amount of genetic progress made in one generation of selection for a quantitative trait depends on ___________________ and ___________________.
124. ______________ is the chief cause of genetic correlation and __________________ is a transient one.

125. ____________________ is the average age of parents when their offspring are born.

126. Phenotype is the interaction of ______________ and ______________.

127. Selection is broadly classified into ____________ and ______________.

128. Hybrid vigor is otherwise known as ________________.

129. Breeder can change the genetic constitution of the population only by ________________ and ________________.

130. ___________ of animal tells us what he seems to be, his ____________ tells us what he ought to be and his ________________ tells us what he is.

131. ___________________ is the most efficient method of selection.

132. Individual selection will be more effective, when heritability of the trait is _____________.

133. ______________ is record of an individual's ancestors.

134. ______________________________ is the basis for the estimation of heritability and genetic correlation.

135. The standardized selection differential is also known as ________________.

136. Corrected daughters' average index was developed by ______________.

137. Santa Gertrudis, a synthetic breed of beef cattle possesses ________________ of Brahman and ________________ of Shorthorn cattle inheritance.

138. The quantitative traits are usually influenced by________________, in addition to genotype.

139. ________________ selection is used for selection of individuals early in life.

140. Family selection is usually practiced in ________________ and ________________ species.

141. ________________ method of selection uses one trait at a time.

142. The information required for construction of selection index are ________________,________________ and __________________.

143. ________________ is the form of family selection that does not include individual record in arriving family mean.

144. Selection is choosing of ________________ for the next generation.

145. Equi-parent index is developed by ________________.

146. Lyre-shaped horns are present in ________________ cattle.

147. Gir is a ________________ breed of cattle and its home tract is ________________ state.

148. The most accurate aid to selection is ________________.

149. Response to selection for quantitative traits is generally less than ________________ as h^2 is usually less than one.

150. The average generation interval in swine is __________ years.

151. A ______________________________ is set for each trait in independent culling method of selection.

152. Rice index is also known as ________________.

153. ________________ selection is not effective when the heritability of a character is low.

154. Regression index = 0.5 (________________) + 0.5 (____________).

155. The value of genetic correlation ranges between ________________ and ________________.

156. Genotype of an animal is fixed at the time of ________________.

157. Tandem method of selection will be useful if the traits considered for selection are ________________ correlated.

158. Individuals whose performance is considered for selection of other individuals, but do not contribute any genes to them are called ________________.

159. Repeatability is the upper limit of ______________, and it includes ________________ environmental variance.

160. ______________ is a English breed of pig originated from Leicester pigs

161. In animal breeding, two animals are said to be related, when they have ________________.

162. A small sized breed of poultry native of Andhra Pradesh is ______________.

163. In small population, the heritability value of a trait will be ________________________ compared to a large random mating population.

164. Principle of construction of selection index is to maximize correlation between ________________ and __________________.

165. Bulls __________________ value is estimated by progeny testing.

166. ___________________ type of gene action is mainly responsible for complementarity.

167. _______________attempts to evaluate the genotype of an animal on the basis of its progeny's performance.

168. The accuracy of selection for a trait is tied directly to its _______________.

169. _________________ has been aptly termed as the key stone of the arch of animal improvement.

170. Crossing zebra and horse produces ________________.

171. A _____________________________ is defined as the one in which selection is primarily for one trait but due to a strong genetic correlation a change occurs in a second trait.

172. The _________________________ refers to the superiority or inferiority, of those selected for parents as compared to the average of the population from which the breeding animals were selected.

173. _________________ and _______________ exotic breeds of sheep contributes fine wool production in the world.

174. _________________ is the exotic breed of dairy cattle originated in English channel used in India for crossbreeding/upgrading.

175. Buffalo with jet black colour is _________________.

176. _________________ is the biggest and majestic breed of goat in India.

177. The MPPA can be expanded as ____________________

178. The time interval between calving and subsequent conception is known as _________________.

179. The native State of Surti breed of buffaloes is ________________.

180. The value of an individual judged by the mean value of its progeny is called _________________.

181. The white colored broiler breed developed in England, which is known for its excellent meat is ________________.

182. Brahman breed belongs to _________________class of poultry.

183. The ratio of selection differential to phenotypic standard deviation of a trait is known as ________________.

184. The exotic breed of pigs extensively used in India for upgrading/ crossbreeding is ________________.

185. The method of selection, which requires the information on relative economic weights and, phenotypic and genetic correlation, is ________________.

186. For improvement of traits with low heritability, ________________ selection aid is more useful.

187. The new breed of dairy cattle evolved in Kerala is ________________.

188. If 'n' traits are considered for selection simultaneously, then the response to selection in each trait decreases at the rate of ________________.

189. The consistency of repetition of same trait several times in the lifetime of an individual is known as ________________.

190. The genetic correlation is the correlation between ________________ of the two traits concerned.

191. Progeny testing is mostly used in selection of ________________ because they produce more progeny in their lifetime.

192. ________________ breed is evolved in Tamil Nadu by crossing Merino and Nilagiri sheep.

193. Heritability of reproductive trait is generally ________________.

194. Egg yield and egg weight are ________________ correlated.

195. The size of the selection differential is otherwise known as ____________ pressure.

196. Geep is the hybrid between ______________ and ________________.

197. ________________ is a new breed of sheep developed at Hisar by crossing Bikaneri ewes and Merino rams.

198. The ratio of ________________ to ________________ is called as coefficient of genetic determination.

199. White leghorn is the most popular bird for its excellent ____________ performance.

200. ______________ an Indian breed of poultry is noted for its majestic gait and dogged fighting qualities.

201. Reciprocal Recurrent Selection involves ________________ inbred line
202. Unmasking of recessive gene occurs in ________________ .
203. Selection Index value = ________________ .
204. Jersind is cross of ________________ ,________________ .
205. Karnah is found in ________________ .
206. h2= R (response to selection)/____________________________ .
207. Genetic basis of Heterosis involves ____________ , ____________ theory.
208. i (intensity of selection) = ______________________________ .
209. Black Bengal is ________________ Breed(sheep/goat
210. Individual selection is used when heritability is _______________ .
211. Heterosis = __________________________________ .
212. Superiority of offspring over average of their parents is ___________ .
213. __________________ is the closest form of inbreeding whereas ________________ is wildest form of out breeding.
214. Limits to selection is due to ________________ .
215. Family selection is done when heritability is ________________ .
216. Frieswal breed of cattle is a cross of __________ and ____________ .
217. The dairy cattle breeds in India are __________ & _____________ .
218. The principal causes of genetic correlation are ________________ & ________________ .
219. The home track of Murrah buffaloes is ________________ and where as that of Vachur cattle are ________________ .
220. The concept of MPPA was given by ________________ where as the concept of heritability was given by ________________ .
221. Buffaloes are mainly of two types: _________________________ & ________________ .
222. Family selection is done when the heritability of a quantitative trait is ___________________________________ .
223. India possesses ________________ number of recognized breeds of cattle and ________________ recognized breeds of buffalo.

224. Genetic improvement per year depends on ____________________ , ________________ & ______________________________.

225. Heritability estimates obtained in full sib correlation are ______________________________ than that obtained in half sib correlation method because presence of ______________________________.

226. Breeding plans comprises of ______________ & _______________ .

227. Inbreeding results in decrease in _________________ accompanied with increase in _______________ in the inbred animals.

228. There is 50% reduction of _____________ in one generation of selfing.

229. Prepotency is the ability of an animal, particularly a sire to ____.

230. Inbred sires are more ______________ because they transmit a given set of characters to their off springs more frequently.

231. Inbreeding coefficient of an animal produced by mating two half sibs is _________________.

232. Inbreeding coefficient of an animal produced by mating sire with its daughter is ___________________.

233. The term coefficient of inbreeding was coined by _______________.

234. Intensity of inbreeding is measured by _______________________.

235. Inbreeding makes a population more variable by producing ______________ .

236. Inbreeding coefficient Fx of an individual X, is given by the formula _________________________.

237. Traits showing heterosis are called often as ___________________.

238. The principle use of inbreeding is to develop ___________________ in _________________________ .

239. Genetic basis of general combining ability and specific combining ability are __________________ and __________________ respectively.

240. Single first cousin have ______________ grand parent in common.

241. ____________ is the closest form of inbreeding whereas ____________ is wildest form of out breeding.

242. The phenomenon of heterosis is due to ________________________ _________ gene action.

KEY

1. Realized
2. Karakul
3. Pulikulam
4. Immediate or recent
5. Denmark
6. Response to selection or Genetic gain
7. Zero
8. Increases
9. Relationship
10. Survival of the fittest
11. Culling
12. Mass selection
13. Genetic correlation
14. Common environmental effect or C^2 effect
15. Sahiwal
16. Hump
17. Intensity of selection
18. Draught
19. *Inter-se*
20. 0 to 1
21. Taylor breed
22. 25 %, 25%
23. Bull or sire or Male
24. Persistency
25. Inbreeding coefficient
26. Mule
27. NBAGR, Karnal
28. Selection and mating or breeding

29. Four breed cross
30. Full sib
31. 45-60 days
32. 50%
33. Line breeding
34. Relationship coefficient, Sewall Wright
35. Inbreeding depression
36. Sterile
37. Lines, line cross
38. Pien niu
39. Nucleus
40. Higher, lower
41. Variation
42. Rambouillet
43. Selection
44. Out
45. Gestation period
46. In
47. Test
48. Inbreeding
49. Incross breeding
50. Outbreeding
51. Back cross
52. Upgrading with Murrah or Surti
53. Line breeding
54. Zero to one
55. Two
56. 365 days
57. Prepotency

58. Malecot
59. 305 days
60. Positive assortative mating
61. Assortative mating
62. 0.25
63. Non additive
64. Out crossing/ selective breeding
65. Heterozygotes
66. Rotational criss crossing
67. Commercial tier/ Farmers' herd
68. Parent offspring
69. Badhawari
70. Hybrid vigour or heterosis
71. 0.50
72. Karan Swiss, Sunandini
73. Selective breeding
74. 0.25
75. European cattle and American Bison
76. *Bos indicus*
77. Murrah
78. Intensity of selection
79. Genes
80. 46.15
81. Regression
82. Crossbreeding, outcrossing
83. Pleiotropy
84. Line breeding
85. Holstein Friesian
86. Progeny testing

87. Rambouillet and Malpura
88. Selection Index
89. Genetically modified organism
90. Mehsana
91. Increases
92. J.L.Lush
93. Hazel
94. Half-sib
95. Linnaeus
96. Selection
97. Best Linear Unbiased Prediction
98. Heritability
99. Standard error
100. Relationship
101. Special and temporary
102. Intra-class correlation
103. Multi-source
104. Non additive
105. G X E interaction
106. One
107. Brown Swiss and Sahiwal
108. Reciprocal recurrent
109. Selection intensity
110. Indirect selection
111. Directly
112. Chicken and elephant
113. Ongole
114. Gene frequency
115. Selection differential, heritability and generation interval

116. New Zealand white and White giant
117. Medium
118. 4 to 4 ½ years
119. Dog
120. Genetic and operational
121. Gene and genotype frequencies
122. Population
123. Selection differential and heritability
124. Pleiotropy, linkage
125. Generation interval
126. Genotype and environment
127. Natural and artificial
128. Heterosis
129. Selection and mating
130. Phenotype, pedigree and progeny
131. Selection index
132. High
133. pedigree
134. Resemblance between relatives
135. Intensity of selection
136. Krishnan's Index
137. 3/8, 5/8
138. Environment
139. Pedigree
140. Swine, poultry
141. Tandom
142. Heritability, genetic correlation and economic value
143. Sib selection
144. Parents

145. Hanson
146. Kankrej
147. Indian/ dairy, Gujarat
148. Progeny testing
149. Selection differential
150. 115
151. Minimum level or culling level
152. Regression index
153. Individual or pedigree
154. Intermediate index, herd average
155. -1 to +1
156. Fertilization
157. Positively
158. Sibs
159. Heritability, Special
160. Yorkshire
161. Common ancestors
162. Kalahasthi
163. Low
164. Index value and true breeding value
165. Breeding
166. Additive
167. Progeny testing
168. Heritability
169. Artificial selection
170. Zebroid
171. Correlated response
172. Selection differential or reach
173. Merino and Rambouillet

174. Jersey
175. Murrah
176. Jamnapari
177. Most Probable Producing Ability
178. Days open / service period
179. Gujarat
180. Breeding value
181. Cornish
182. Asiatic
183. Intensity of selection
184. Large white Yarkshire
185. Selection Index
186. Progeny testing
187. Sunandini
188. 1/ Ön
189. Repeatability
190. Breeding value
191. Bulls or males
192. Sandyno
193. Low
194. Negatively
195. Selection
196. Goat and sheep
197. Hissardale
198. $V_{G'}$ V_P
199. Egg production
200. Aseel
201. Zero
202. Inbreeding

203. Heritability x economic traits
204. Jersey and Red sindhi
205. Kashmir
206. Selection Differencial
207. Dominance, over dominance
208. z/p
209. goat
210. high
211. mean of F1 progeny - mean of parental breed
212. heterosis
213. self-fertilization, species hybridization
214. exhaustion of genetic variance
215. low
216. Friesian, Sahiwal
217. Sahiwal, Red Sindhi.
218. Linkage, Pleotropy
219. Haryana, Karala
220. Lush, Lush
221. Reverine, Swamp
222. Low
223. 30, 8
224. Intensity of selection, heritability, Phenotypic Std. Deviation
225. Higher, Maternal effect
226. Matting, Selection
227. Heterozygosity, Homozygosity
228. Heterozygosity
229. Stamp its characteristic on progeny
230. Prepotent
231. 0.125

232. 0.25
233. Sewell Wright
234. Inbreeding Co-efficient
235. Inbreed lines
236.
237. Heterotic trait
238. Inbreed lines ; Poultry
239. additive gene action ; Non- additive gene action
240. Two
241. Selfing ; species hybridization
242. Non-Additive

2. State True or False

1. Environmental variations reduce the accuracy of selection in genetic studies.
2. Survival of the fittest is the basic principle operating under natural selection
3. Diallele crossing is commonly practiced in cattle.
4. Highest contribution to total milk production in India is from buffaloes.
5. Genetic gain is directly proportional to the selection intensity.
6. Response to selection is very poor when the number of animals selected in a genetic improvement programme is high.
7. Amrithmahal is a dual purpose breed of cattle.
8. Progeny testing is for the selection of off-springs
9. The heterosis of the F_2 will always be more than F_1 generation
10. Inbreeding can be avoided in a farm by planned selection and mating using the breeding records
11. For traits which are sex limited and expressed later stage in life, pedigree selection can be practiced
12. The increase in the age at first calving decreases the generation interval in bull production program

13. Out breeding increases the heterozygosity in the population
14. In dairy cattle maximum genetic improvement is brought by the male selection than by female selection
15. *In-situ* conservation involves the maintenance of live population of animals in their home tract.
16. According to Shaler (1985), dog was the first animal domesticated
17. Recurrent and reciprocal recurrent selection methods are commonly used in cattle improvement programs
18. Mongrel is a crossbred that is unacceptable or unplanned.
19. Mehsana is the buffalo produced by crossing Murrah and Surti.
20. In CNBS selection of males and females is done at the commercial tier also
21. Inbreeding increases prepotency
22. In ONBS, the nucleus herd is constituted by the genetically superior animals
23. In CNBS, nucleus tier consists of 30-40% of the population
24. Grading up is the form of inbreeding where animals belonging to two different breeds are mated
25. Open nucleus breeding scheme is used for cattle and buffalo genetic improvement
26. Complementarity is due to non-additive gene action while heterosis is due to additive gene action
27. Improvement of milk production potential of buffaloes in India can be achieved by cross breeding with exotic animals
28. Non-additive genetic variance is the chief cause of resemblance between relatives
29. In pedigree selection of an individual, the recent ancestor should receive most emphasis than the distant ancestors
30. Grading up is the form of out breeding in which same sire of one pure breed is used on the females of non-descript animals.
31. Close inbreeding is done to develop inbred lines with relatively higher degree of homozygosity at a faster rate.
32. Increasing of homozygosity through inbreeding is the only way of increasing the prepotency.

33. Repeatability sets an upper limit to heritability of a trait.
34. The intra-sire regression of offspring on dam estimate is equal to ½ h^2
35. The keystone of arch of Animal Breeding is selection.
36. Family selection is useful for traits of low heritability.
37. The heritability value estimated for a population cannot be applied for another.
38. Covariance of full sibs is equal to ½ of V_A.
39. Use of old bulls decreases generation interval.
40. Genetic gain is more in an expanding herd.
41. Polygenes are responsible for genetic correlation.
42. If repeated measures on the same animal are similar to each other, the trait is said to be lowly repeatable.
43. Bias in the estimate of heritability is introduced by environmental source of covariance and variance due to dominance.
44. Indirect selection can be of use where the two traits are highly genetically correlated, and the secondary trait is highly heritable.
45. In general, the characters closely connected with reproductive fitness are highly heritable.
46. Family selection will be successful if the number of progeny in each family is large.
47. Mass selection is not effective when the heritability of the trait is high.
48. When heritability of a trait is high, heterosis for the trait is also high.
49. The advantage of index method of selection increases with the number of traits included in the index.
50. There is possibility of increase in inbreeding in family selection.
51. Inbred lines are produced by mating among related individuals in a closed flock.
52. Diallele crossing is a method of progeny testing for selecting strains / lines for crossing to exploit heterosis.
53. The term reach is used to indicate the phenotypic superiority of selected parents over the population mean.
54. Ongole is the best Indian milch breed of cattle.

55. Genetic variability within a population is necessary if selection is to be effective over a long period of time.
56. Individual selection is not possible in both sexes for sex limited traits.
57. Progeny testing is more accurate than individual selection when the heritability of the trait is low.
58. Heritability decreases with inbreeding and increases with outcrossing.
59. Lesser the variance among the individuals more will be the selection differential.
60. Higher selection differential results in higher genetic gain.
61. Variation between the phenotype of monozygotic twins is wholly environmental in origin.
62. A single population that is a mixture of genes from various populations is called a synthetic.
63. Selection differential is not influenced by the sex of the individual.
64. Heritability and repeatability estimates for fertility traits in dairy cattle are very high.
65. Multiple ovulation and embryo transfer technique would reduce generation interval.
66. Calving interval is the sum of gestation period and dry period.
67. The selection differential is higher when smaller proportion of individuals is selected in a population.
68. Phenotypic selection will be more effective for traits with low heritability.
69. Males have more selection differential than females.
70. Pedigree selection is not useful for sex-limited traits.
71. Most of the economic traits are generally controlled by few or major genes.
72. Phenotype is a good indicator of genotype only when the variations are largely due to non-genetic differences.
73. Heritability is the ratio between additive and non-additive genetic variances.
74. The standard lactation length in dairy cattle is 305 days.
75. Standardized selection differential is known as response.

76. Dorset is an indigenous sheep breed of Himachal Pradesh.
77. Expression of quantitative traits is generally influenced by environment.
78. Selection is the choosing of parents for next generation.
79. Repeatability indicates how much of the superiority of parents is expressed in their progeny.
80. Milk yield and fat per cent are positively correlated traits.
81. The ratio of genetic gain and selection differential is known as realized heritability.
82. The annual genetic gain increases as the generation interval increases.
83. Heritability is the regression of breeding value on phenotypic value.
84. Tandem method of selection is not applicable for negatively correlated traits.
85. Equi-parent index is also known as Yapp's index.
86. Sunandini is a dairy purpose cattle developed in Kerala.
87. The genetic correlation ranges from zero to one.
88. Recurrent selection improves the GCA of tester line and SCA of the line cross simultaneously.
89. The lyre-shaped horns are present in Kankrej breed of cattle.
90. Heritability of the fitness and survivability traits is high.
91. Progeny testing is the best way of determining the breeding value of an individual.
92. Toda buffalo is reared by the tribal people in the Nilgiri district of Tamil Nadu.
93. Most of the economic traits are governed by many genes and are greatly influenced by environment.
94. Family selection is commonly used in poultry and swine.
95. Jersey is an exotic dairy cattle breed.
96. Individual selection is also known as mass selection.
97. Correlated response is high, when the traits are unrelated.
98. Phenotype is the genetic constitution of an individual.
99. Pedigree selection is easier and cheaper to perform.

100. Response to selection is less than or equal to selection differential and never be higher than selection differential.

101. The first herd book was started for Shorthorn cattle.

102. Closed herd book allows the entry of individuals, which have registered ancestry or certain specific breed requirements.

103. The regression of offspring on mid-parent is equal to heritability.

104. Individual selection is applied for sex-limited traits.

105. The record of descendants is known as pedigree.

106. In individual selection, the square root of heritability is known as accuracy of selection.

107. Tandem method of selection is preferred only for traits having desirable genetic correlation.

108. Resemblance between relatives is the basis for estimation of repeatability.

109. Independent culling method of selection is most efficient among all methods of selection.

110. The repeatability ranges between zero and one.

111. Construction of selection index is relatively simple.

112. Progeny testing is applied for improvement of carcass traits.

113. The higher common environmental effect among the members of the family affects the accuracy of family selection.

114. Generation interval in sheep is usually 4 - 4½ years.

115. V_G is partitioned into V_P and V_E.

116. Hariana is a dual purpose cattle breed of India.

117. The optimum dry period in dairy cattle is 45 - 60 days.

118. The value of an individual judged by mean value of its progeny is known as breeding value.

119. The genus of exotic cattle is *taurus*.

120. The recurrent selection method for improving the combining ability was proposed by Hull.

121. Objective traits are visual appraisal traits.

122. Use of young bulls increases generation interval.

123. Phenotypic variation is completely due to differences in genes.

124. Hinny is the hybrid obtained by crossing mare with Jackass.

125. Environmental variation common to the members of a family improves the efficiency of family selection.

126. Response to selection depends on selection intensity.

127. Reciprocal recurrent selection is a method of progeny testing.

128. Specific combining ability is for a line or breed and general combining ability is for a cross.

129. Response to selection is more for traits primarily controlled by additive genes.

130. Heritability is an individual's measure.

131. Swine are known as " Mortgage lifters".

132. Sahiwal is one of the best Indian milch breeds.

133. Pashmina is produced by sheep.

134. Heritability estimation in cattle is usually done by paternal half sib analysis method.

135. Effectiveness of selection on the basis of phenotype will be high when h^2 is low.

136. As the generation interval increases, the genetic gain per annum will also increase.

137. Natural selection eliminates unsuccessful combinations and allows only the successful combinations to multiply.

138. Non-additive gene action tends to increase the heritability.

139. Repeatability is measured for traits expressed several times during an animal's lifetime.

140. Removing less productive animals from the population is called selection.

141. Breed type characters should be given much importance during selection for milk yield.

142. Selection will be effective if foundation animals have no genetic diversity.

143. Pedigree could alone be used as a major aid in selection.

144. Pullikulam breed of cattle is otherwise called as Jallikattu.

145. Because an animal passes only half of its genes to its progeny, it passes on only half its breeding value.
146. Piglets of the same litter are said to be half- sibs.
147. Mating American Bison with domestic cattle produces as Cattalo.
148. Linkage is a cause for environmental correlation.
149. Positive assortative mating increases heritability.
150. When heritability of a trait is more, the accuracy of individual selection is more.
151. Independent culling level method of selection gives due weightage to heritability of the trait.
152. Asiatic breeds of poultry have feathered shanks.
153. Assel is the indigenous breed of poultry known for high stamina, majestic gait and dogged fighting qualities
154. The pelt (fur) producing sheep breed is Karakul
155. The Anglo Nubian is known as the jersey of goat breeds
156. The milk queen of goat world is Sannen
157. The breed of buffaloe producing milk with highest fat percentage is Bhadawari
158. The father of modern animal breeding is Robert Bakewell
159. The shorthorn breed of cattle was developed by Robert Bakewell
160. Genetic correlation is defined as the correlation between the breeding values of the traits
161. Recurrent selection is proposed by Hull.
162. Breeding Strategies involves selection and mating system.
163. Population of endangered breed is more.
164. Double hump camel is not under threat of extinction.
165. Progeny testing is based on the sampling nature of inheritance.
166. Heterosis depends on the occurrence of dominance loci.
167. Mating of unrelated individual is called in breeding
168. Rambouillet is a sheep breed.

169. Line breeding is a type of outbreeding.
170. Heritability time's phenotypic value is equal to breeding value of the animal for a particular trait.
171. Heritability is the upper limit of repeatability.
172. Individual selection is practiced when h2 of the trait is low.
173. Selection Differential is the difference in the mean performance of selected individuals and the mean of their progeny
174. Selection is not a differential reproduction.
175. Genetic basis of General combining ability is non-additive gene action.
176. Specific combining ability of a cross is due to heterotic effects of genes.
177. In Truncation selection there is clear-cut demarcation between selected and rejected individuals for further breeding.
178. Indirect selection is practiced to take the benefit of correlated response.
179. Barberi is a sheep breed of India.
180. Repeatability is upper limit of heritability.
181. When the repeatability of a tract is high, the animal with poor performance could be culled at an early age.
182. Repeatability of most of the production traits is very low because they are least influenced by non-genetic factors.
183. Indirect selection is practiced to take the benefit of correlated response.
184. By taking multiple measurements, additive genetic variance gets reduced.
185. Covariance of full sibs measures one fourth of additive genetic variance.
186. Half sib correlation method is the best method for estimating repeatability of a quantitative trait.
187. Quantitative traits are least influenced by non-genetic factors.
188. Breeding value of an animal is equal to its transmitting ability.
189. Barberi is a Dairy Goat breed of India.
190. Breeding tract of buffaloes of Murrah breed is the state of Rajasthan.
191. Covariance of half sibs measures one fourth of additive genetic variance.
192. Progeny testing results are expressed in the form of selection indices.

193. Heritability time's phenotypic value is equal to breeding value of the animal for a particular trait.
194. Heritability is the upper limit of repeatability.
195. Individual selection is practiced when h2 of the trait is low.
196. Selection Differential is the difference in the mean performance of selected individuals and the mean of their progeny
197. Indirect selection can give faster improvement than does the direct selection when the genetic correlation between the two traits is high.
198. Genetic basis of General combining ability is non-additive gene action.
199. Specific combining ability of a cross is due to heterotic effects of genes.
200. In Truncation selection there is clear-cut demarcation between selected and rejected individuals for further breeding.
201. Inbreeding coefficient of an individual from full sib mating is 0.125.
202. Consequences of Inbreeding and genetic assortative mating are not same.
203. Formula for coefficient of relationship was given by R. A. Fisher.
204. Two individuals having same inbreeding coefficient will be homozygous at the same loci.
205. Inbreeding increases the total variability in the population.
206. Out-breeding is mating of animals outside the herd.
207. Inbreeding changes gene and genotype frequency.
208. The species hybrid produced from the mating of stallion and a female ass is called as mule.
209. In case of Open Nucleus Breeding System, the replacement males & females of the nucleus are generated from the nucleus only.
210. Incase of Open Nucleus Breeding System the gene flow from outside is not allowed into the nucleus.
211. Upgrading system of mating changes the genetic composition by creating new genes
212. Species hybridization is the widest possible type out breeding
213. Jatsa produces from crossing of Mithun and Cow are F1 females
214. Crossbreeding is effective for traits that can not be improved by selection with a breed due to less genetic variability.

215. Top crossing is a form of inbreeding and is like grading up system
216. Criss-crossing involves three established breeds.
217. Species hybrids are mostly sterile.
218. If two individuals A & B are two double first cousins, they must have four grand parents in common.
219. Survival and fertility are the two main characters associated with natural fitness and are affected under inbreeding.
220. Cross breeding increases homozygosity where as inbreeding increases heterozygocity.

KEY

1.	True	2.	True
3.	False	4.	True
5.	True	6.	True
7.	False	8.	False
9.	False	10.	True
11.	True	12.	False
13.	True	14.	True
15.	True	16.	True
17.	False	18.	True
19.	True	20.	False
21.	True	22.	True
23.	False	24.	False
25.	True	26.	False
27.	False	28.	False
29.	True	30.	False
31.	True	32.	True
33.	True	34.	True
35.	True	36.	True
37.	True	38.	True
39.	False	40.	True
41.	True	42.	False
43.	True	44.	True

45.	False	46.	True
47.	False	48.	False
49.	False	50.	True
51.	True	52.	True
53.	True	54.	False
55.	True	56.	True
57.	True	58.	True
59.	False	60.	True
61.	True	62.	True
63.	False	64.	False
65.	True	66.	False
67.	True	68.	False
69.	True	70.	False
71.	False	72.	False
73.	False	74.	True
75.	False	76.	False
77.	True	78.	True
79.	False	80.	False
81.	True	82.	False
83.	True	84.	True
85.	True	86.	False
87.	False	88.	True
89.	True	90.	False
91.	True	92.	True
93.	True	94.	True
95.	True	96.	True
97.	False	98.	False
99.	True	100.	True
101.	True	102.	True
103.	True	104.	False
105.	False	106.	True
107.	True	108.	False
109.	False	110.	True

111. False
112. True
113. True
114. False
115. False
116. True
117. True
118. True
119. True
120. True
121. True
122. False
123. False
124. False
125. False
126. True
127. True
128. False
129. True
130. False
131. True
132. True
133. False
134. True
135. False
136. False
137. True
138. False
139. True
140. False
141. False
142. False
143. False
144. True
145. True
146. False
147. True
148. False
149. False
150. True
151. False
152. True
153. True
154. True
155. True
156. True
157. True
158. False
159. False
160. True
161. True
162. True
163. False
164. False
165. True
166. True
167. False
168. True
169. False
170. True
171. False
172. False
173. False
174. False
175. False
176. True

177. True
178. True
179. False
180. True
181. True
182. False
183. True
184. False
185. True
186. False
187. False
188. False
189. True
190. False
191. True
192. False
193. False
194. False
195. False
196. False
197. True
198. False
199. True
200. True
201. False
202. False
203. True
204. False
205. False
206. False
207. False
208. False
209. False
210. False
211. False
212. True
213. False
214. True
215. False
216. False
217. True
218. True
219. True
220. False

3. Choose the Most Appropriate Answer

1. Sahiwal is classified as
   a) Dual purpose breed
   b) Dairy breed
   c) Draught breed
   d) None of the above

2. Gir cattle are native of
   a) Rajasthan
   b) Hariana
   c) Gujarat
   d) West Bengal

3. Most efficient method of selection is
   a) Index selection
   b) Tandem method
   c) Independent culling method
   d) Progeny testing

4. Herd book was first started for

   a) Horse b) Cattle
   c) Sheep e) None of the above

5. Choosing of parents for next generation is known as

   a) Selection b) Culling
   c) Breeding d) Mating

6. Heritability in broad sense is

   a) V_A/V_P b) V_G/V_P
   c) V_E/V_P d) None of the above

7. Karan-Swiss and Karan-Fries cattle were developed in

   a) NDRI, Karnal b) IVRI, Izatnagar
   c) PDC, Meerut d) CSWRI, Avika Nagar

8. The sib selection is a type of

   a) Progeny testing b) Pedigree selection
   c) Family selection d) None of the above

9. Generation interval in cattle is

   a) 2 to 2 1/2 Years b) 4 to 4 1/2 Years
   c) 6 to 6 1/2 Years d) None of the above

10. Dairy search index is otherwise called as

    a) Sunderasan index b) Tomer index
    c) Rice index d) Krishnan Index

11. Malecot's method of calculating coefficient of relationship is otherwise called

    a) Variance-covariance chart b) Variance ratio method
    c) Over dominance chart d) Standard ratio method

12. The humped cattle of India and Pakistan are known as

    a) Zebu b) Teghu
    c) Khehu d) Chegu

13. Mating of small bull to small cow is known as

a) Random mating
b) Negative Assortative mating
c) Positive assortative mating
d) Panmixia

14. Father of animal breeding

a) S.Wright
b) J.L. Lush
c) Charles Darwin
d) Robert Bakewell

15. The coefficient of inbreeding of the progeny born out of full sib mating is

a) 50 %
b) 12.5%
c) 25%
d) 100%

16. The interval between calving and subsequent conception is known as

a) Calving interval
b) Dry period
c) Days open
d) Conception rate

17. All the factors affecting the performance or expression of a trait that are not due to the genes are called as

a) Non-additive gene action
b) Additive gene action
c) Dominance
d) Environment

18. Rotational crossing is suitable for the improvement of

a) Horses
b) Pigs
c) Cattle
d) Dogs

19. According to Shaler (1985) the first animal domesticated was

a) Horse
b) Dog
c) Elephant
d) Sheep

20. Inbreeding is the mating of related individuals within

a) 4-6 generations
b) 5-7 generations
c) 7-8 generations
d) 7-9 generations

21. The Australian Milking Zebu is a cross between

a) Friesian and Sahiwal
b) Jersey and Friesian
c) Jersey and Tharparkar
d) Jersey and Sahiwal

22. Mating of large bull to small cow is known as

a) Random mating b) Negative Assortative mating

c) Positive assortative mating d) Panmixia

23. The coefficient of inbreeding of the progeny born out of full sib mating is

a) 50 % b) 12.5%

c) 25% d) 100%

24. Heterosis is F1 generation is equal to

a) Ó dy2 b) Ó d2y2

c) Ó dy3 d) Ó d2y

25. Mating of an outstanding sire to its female progenies in successive generations is known as

a) Out crossing b) Line crossing

c) Line breeding d) Backward mating

26. The interval between two successive calving is known as

a) Calving interval b) Dry period

c) Days open d) Conception rate

27. The coefficient of relationship ranges from

a) $-\mu$ to $+\mu$ b) 0 to μ

c) -1 to $+1$ d) 0 to 1

28. Inbreeding is useful to

a) Eliminate the undesirable genes
b) Develop inbred lines
c) Develop new breeds of livestock
d) All of the above

29. Average age of the parent when the offspring is born is

a) Genetic gain per year b) Generation interval

c) Age at birth d) None of the above

30. The increased level of performance of progenies as compared to the average of the parental types is known as

a) Heterosis b) Inbreeding depression

c) Selection differential d) Prepotency

31. The weaning of piglet is done at the age of

a) 90 days
b) 180 days
c) 120 days
d) 56 days

32. Out breeding is done

a) To exploit heterosis
b) To introduce new genes
c) To produce commercial animals
d) All the above

33. Specific combining ability is practiced to take the advantage of

a) Genotype environmental interaction
b) Additive gene action
c) Non additive gene action
d) All the above

34. Family selection will be more effective than the individual selection for

a) Low heritable traits
b) Highly heritable traits
c) Both a and b
d) None of the above

35. Qualities needed for an individual to have more prepotency are

a) High per cent of dominant genes
b) Higher homozygosity
c) Both a and b
d) None of the above

36. In buffaloes, the breed that requires conservation is

a) Toda
b) Surti
c) Murrah
d) Gir

37. Mass selection is more effective if the heritability of the trait is

a) Low
b) Medium
c) High
d) Negative

38. Pedigree selection is more effective when heritability of the trait is

a) Low
b) High
c) Zero
d) None of the above

39. Selection that cannot be used for sex-limited traits is

a) Progeny selection | b) Pedigree selection
c) Individual selection | d) None of the above

40. Heritability in narrow sense is

a) V_A/V_P | b) V_G/V_P
c) V_E/V_P | d) $V_G + V_E / V_P$

41. The crossbred cattle developed at PDC, Meerut is

a) Karan Swiss | b) Taylor breed
c) Frieswal | d) Sunandini

42. Brangus cattle was developed by crossing Brahman cattle with

a) Shorthorn | b) Brown-Swiss
c) Angus | d) None of the above

43. Selection differential is equal to

a) i/s_P | b) i/s_P^2
c) is_P | d) None of the above

44. The coefficient never lower than the coefficient of genetic determination is

a) Repeatability | b) Heritability
c) Genetic correlation | d) None of the above

45. The process that increases the frequency of desirable genes without creating or introducing new one is known as

a) Crossbreeding | b) Inbreeding
c) Selection | d) None of these

46. The breed of cattle which has high milk production and low fat per cent is

a) Jersey | b) Holstein Friesian
c) Brown Swiss | d) Sahiwal

47. The habitat of Kankrej cattle is

a) Rann of Kutch | b) Sind Province
c) Punjab | d) Karnataka

48. The sire index that includes contemporary performance is

a) Equi parent index b) Dairy search index
c) Krishnan index d) Yapp index

49. Genetic correlation between milk yield and fat per cent is

a) Positive b) Zero
c) Negative d) Two

50. In cattle the 'lyre' shaped horn is present in

a) Ongole b) Kankrej
c) Umblachery d) Jersey

51. If two traits "A" and "B" are negatively correlated, then as "A" improves, "B" will

a) Increase b) Decrease
c) Remain unchanged d) Double

52. In independent culling method of selection, if very high standards are fixed, the number of animals selected to become parents will be

a) Very large b) Very small
c) Moderate d) None of the above

53. By selection on the basis of progeny, we can know what an

a) Individual seems to be b) Individual ought to be
c) Individual is d) None of the above

54. An example of draught breed of cattle is

a) Gir b) Red Sindhi
c) Hallikar d) Sahiwal

55. The exotic breed of pig widely used for upgrading the desi pigs is

a) Large White Yorkshire b) Berkshire
c) Landrace d) Soviet Chinchilla

56. The home tract of Jamnapari goat is in

a) Kerala state b) Uttar Pradesh state
c) Maharashtra state d) Jammu & Kashmir

57. The indigenous breed of dairy cattle which is called as White Sindhi

a) Ongole
b) Sahiwal
c) Tharparkar
d) Red Sindhi

58. Culling can be practiced with few records if the repeatability of the trait is

a) Low
b) High
c) Medium
d) Zero

59. Recurrent selection is used to exploit the effect of

a) Additive gene action
b) Non-additive gene action
c) G x E interaction
d) None of the above

60. An individual receives

a) No genes from collateral relatives
b) Half of the genes from collateral relatives
c) One third of the genes from collateral relatives
d) None of the above

61. Independent culling method is

a) Superior to tandem method
b) Inferior to tandem method
c) Superior to selection index method
d) Similar to tandem method

62. In individual selection, animals are chosen on the basis of their

a) Progeny's performance
b) Pedigree
c) Own phenotype
d) Parents performance

63. The efficiency of selection is very low in

a) Tandem method
b) Selection index method
c) Independent culling method
d) None of the above

64. Corrected daughter average index is

a) Rice index
b) Krishnan index
c) Yapp index
d) None of the above

65. Hallikar is a

a) Dairy breed
b) Dual purpose breed
c) Draught breed
d) None of the above

66. The most accurate aid to selection is

a) Individual selection
b) Progeny testing
c) Pedigree selection
d) None of the above

67. The average generation interval in sheep is

a) 9 to13 years
b) 4 to 4 1/2 years
c) 1 to 1/2 years
d) None of the above

68. Animals failing to meet the minimum standard for a trait are culled in

a) Independent culling method
b) Tandem method
c) Selection index method
d) None of the above

69. The genetic correlation between egg production and egg weight is generally

a) Positive
b) Zero
c) Negative
d) None of the above

70. Large White Yorkshire breed of pigs is native of

a) China
b) United States
c) Northern England
d) None of the above

71. The famous dual purpose cattle breed of Andhra pradesh is

a) Sahiwal
b) Kankrej
c) Ongole
d) None of the above

72. The value of an individual judged by the mean value of its offspring is

a) Breeding value
b) Phenotypic value
c) Non-additive genetic value
d) None of the above

73. Sandyno breed is evolved by crossing

a) Merino x Nilagiri
b) Rambouillet x Chokla
c) Dorset x Nilagiri
d) Merino x Nali

74. Dairy Search Index was developed at
    a) NDRI b) IVRI
    c) NDDB d) CSWRI

75. Repeatability of a trait increases when
    a) V_P increases b) V_{ET} increases
    c) V_{EP} increases d) V_G decreases

76. Two individuals will be alike in
    a) Fraternal twins b) Maternal twins
    c) Identical twins d) Full-sibs

77. Mass selection is applicable for
    a) Sex-limited traits b) Traits expressed late in life
    c) Traits with high h^2 d) All of the above

78. The breed of goat considered as most prolific is
    a) Jamunapari b) Barbari
    c) Black Bengal d) Beetal

79. Milch breed of cattle
    a) Hariana b) Ongole
    c) Sahiwal d) Amrithmahal

80. Reciprocal recurrent selection is most suitable for
    a) Cattle b) Sheep
    c) Horse d) Poultry

81. Heritability estimate ranges from
    a) –1 to +1 b) 0 to +1
    c) –1 to 0 d) None of the above

82. The most recent method of sire evaluation is
    a) Contemporary comparison b) Herd-mate comparison
    c) BLUP d) Animal model

83. Selection differential depends upon

a) Proportion of animal selected
b) Variance of the trait
c) Both a and b
d) None of these

84. Superior carpet wool breed of Indian sheep is

a) Chokla b) Deccani
c) Hassan d) All the above

85. To increase the milk production of the indigenous dairy cattle, most suitable breed is

a) Brown Swiss b) Danish
c) Holstein-Friesian d) Boer

86. If a trait is largely controlled by environment, heritability estimate shall be

a) High b) Low
c) Medium d) One

87. Most effective aid to selection for improvement of a sex-limited trait is

a) Sib-selection b) Progeny testing
c) Family seletion d) None of the above

88. Karan-Swiss is the cross between

a) HF and Brown-Swiss b) HF and Sahiwal
c) Brown -Swiss and Sahiwal d) Brown-Swiss and Gir

89. Genetic correlation ranges from

a) 0 to 1 b) –1 to 0
c) –1 to +1 d) 0 to á

90. Heritability estimate in a inbred population will be

a) High b) Low
c) One d) Negative

91. Maximum production from the livestock can be obtained from
    a) Superior herd with poor environment
    b) Superior genotype with best environment
    c) Poor genotype with best environment
    d) Poor genotype with poor environment

92. Merino and Leghorn are developed in
    a) Switzerland   b) England
    c) Spain   d) U.S.A

93. A temperate Himalayan breed of sheep is
    a) Bikaneri   b) Gaddi
    c) Marwari   d) Nilgiri

94. A buffalo breed developed by crossing Murrah and Surti is
    a) Godavari   b) Bhadawari
    c) Jaffarabadi   d) Mehsana

95. If all the individuals in the population are selected as parents then the selection differential will be
    a) 1.00   b) 100 per cent
    c) Infinite   d) Zero

96. The unit of selection in family selection is
    a) Individuals' performance   b) Family mean
    c) Pedigree information   d) Within family deviation

97. The breed of sheep valued for its fur pelt is
    a) Merino   b) Rambouillet
    c) Karakul   d) Corriedale

98. The Rhode Island Red belongs to
    a) American class   b) Mediterranean class
    c) English class   d) Asiatic class

99. The ideal dry period in dairy cattle is
    a) 45-60 days   b) 120-180 days
    c) 240-360 days   d) 480-720 days

100. Genetic gain per year depends on

a) Dry period
b) Calving interval
c) Generation interval
d) Lactation length

101. The native country of Jersey breed is

a) England
b) Germany
c) Russia
d) Australia

102. The Rambouillet breed of sheep is from

a) England
b) Germany
c) USA
d) France

103. Carcass quality is best estimated by

a) Recent ancestors
b) Individual information
c) Sib testing
d) All the above

104. Individuals born in the same period, season and same herd are called

a) Contemporaries
b) Twins
c) Collateral relatives
d) None of these

105. Genetic gain increases with

a) Increased variation in the population
b) Reduced selection differential
c) Reduced heritability
d) Increased generation interval

106. In mass selection, genotype is estimated on the basis of

a) Sibs
b) Ancestors
c) Own phenotype
d) None of these

107. Genetic correlation between body weight an growth rate is

a) Positive
b) Negative
c) Zero
d) None of these

108. The correlation between repeated measurements in the same animal is termed as

a) Correlation
b) Repeatability
c) Linkage
d) Heritability

109. The animals can be selected for show purpose

a) Based on its phenotype
b) Based on its genotype
c) Based on its relatives
d) Based on its pedigree information

110. Selection is efficient in improvement of economic traits since it

a) Create new genes
b) Increases the frequencies of desirable genes
c) Increases favourable environment
d) None of these

111. High heritability indicates high correlation between

a) Genotype and phenotype
b) Genotype and environment
c) Phenotype and environment
d) All of them

112. Most of the economic traits are

a) Controlled by many genes and are greatly influenced by the environment
b) Controlled by a few pairs of genes and not influenced by environment
c) Controlled by many genes and not influenced by environment
d) None of these

113. The breed of Indian goat originated in Asia Minor (Turkey) is

a) Boer
b) Toggenberg
c) Angoa
d) None of the above

114. The native state of Deoni breed is

a) Tamil Nadu
b) Maharashtra
c) Madhya Pradesh
d) None of these

115. The phenotype is a good indicator of the genotype when the heritability of a character is

a) Low
b) High
c) Moderate
d) Zero

116. Which of the following is correct? The repeatability of a trait is:

a) A higher limit for the value of heritability
b) Used to predict MPPA
c) Used to predict future performance from past records
d) All of the above

117. Progeny testing is more valuable than mass selection because

a) Generation interval is increased
b) Accuracy of estimating breeding value can be increased
c) It can be used for lowly heritable traits
d) Both b) and c)

118. Which of the following is incorrect?. The selection intensity

a) Depends on the heritability
b) Can be different for males and females
c) Is higher when fewer animals are selected
d) None of the above

119. In Deccani sheep, the selection differential for 6 months body weight is 3 kg and response to selection is 1.2 kg then the realized heritability for the trait will be

a) 0.4
b) 0.48
c) 0.6
d) None of the above

120. Identify the cattle which does not belong to the group of 'Mysore breeds'

a) Kangayam
b) Ongole
c) Hallikar
d) Alambadi

121. Breed of buffalo capable of surviving in high altitude is

a) Murrah
b) Toda
c) Surti
d) Nagpuri

122. The reduction of hybridvigor in F_2 generation compared to F_1 is expected to be

a) 100%
b) 50%
c) 25%
d) None of the above

123. Change in breeding value expected per unit change in phenotypic value is called

a) Repeatability b) Selection
c) Heritability d) Genetic Correlation

124. Theoretically, if environmental variance is nil, heritability in broad sense is equal to

a) +1 b) -1
c) Zero d) Infinity

125. The estimate that attempts to express what a sire would have produced had he been a cow

a) Progeny Testing b) Selection Index
c) Sire index d) Sire variance

126. Which of the following breeds doesn't come under group of Gujarath buffaloes

a) Mehsana b) Surti
c) Murrah d) Jafferabadi

127. Which of the following cattle breed is not a native of Rajesthan

a) Tharparkar b) Nagori
c) Rathi d) Bargur

128. Which of the following sheep breed is not from north temperate zone

a) Bhakarwal b) Rampur Bushair
c) Nilgiri d) Gaddi

129. Superiority of selected parents over the population is

a) Response to selection b) Selection differential
c) Intensity of selection d) Accuracy of selection

130. Which of the following is the best method of selection for milk yield and fat% content of milk

a) Tandem method b) Independent culling level
c) Selection index d) None of the above

131. According to the latest breeding policy of cattle and buffaloes, which of the following breeds can be used for genetic improvement of cattle?

a. Jersey and Holstein Friesian
b. Jersey and Brown Swiss
c. Holstein Friesian and Brown Swiss
d. Holstein Friesian alone

132. Which of the following is most economical way to introduce genes to a population?

a) Line breeding
b. Cross breeding
c) Species hybridization
d. Inbreeding

133. Which of the following is the wildest form of mating?

a) Upgrading
b) Cross breeding
c) Species hybridization
d) Inbreeding

134. If the average performance of the progenies of a pair of animals exceed the average performance of its parents, the condition is

a) Overdominance
b. Heterosis
c. Inbreeding depression
d. None of the above

135. The probability of genes at a locus in an animal to be identical by descent

a) Coefficient of inbreeding
b) Coefficient of coancestry
c) Coefficient of kinship
d) All of the above

136. Which of the following is a form of inbreeding

a) Incrossbreeding
b) Line breeding
c) Outcrossing
d) Species hybridisation

137. Which of the following is not a crossbred

a) Brangus
b) Bharath Merino
c) Avikalin
d) Catello

138. The National Bureau of Animal Genetic Resources is situated in

a) New Delhi
b) Karnal
c) Hyderabad
d) None of the three

139. Sundanhini is a

a) Brown Swiss crossbred of Kerala
b) Jersey crossbred of Kerala
c) Holstein crossbred of Kerala
d) Crossbred of Tamil Nadu

140. Which of the following is not involved in production of heterosis?

a) Dominance
b) Over dominance
c) Additive gene action
d) Non additive gene action

141. Inbreeding co-efficient range from

a. 1-2
b. 0-1
c. 1-5
d. None

142. Application of Inbreeding

a. Elimination of undesirable gene
b. It produces inbred line
c. Increases prepotency
d. All

143. Selection is ______________ reproduction.

a. Deferential
b. Detrimental
c. Declined
d. All

144. Inbreeding

a. Increases homozygosity
b. Decreases heterozygosity
c. Both
d. Either
e. None

145. Upgrading is

a. Inbreeding
b. Out breeding
c. Both

146. Individual Selection is done when

a. h2 is high
b. h2 is less
c. Both
d. One

147. Pedigree Selection is preferred for traits of

a. High h2 | b. Low h2
c. Both | d. None

148. Inter-se mating is

a. Unlike—like mating | b. Like—like mating
c. Like —unlike mating | d. None

149. Mule is cross of

a. Jack x Mare | b. Cattle x buffalo
c. Cattle x yak | d. None

150. Changthangi is found in

a. Ladakh region of J&K | b Rajouri region of J& K
c. Poonch region of J&K | d. None

151. The following is not a dairy breed of cattle

a) Gir | b) Hariana
c) Sahiwal | d) Red sindhi

152. The following is not the criteria for breed classification

a) Geographical distribution | b) Morphological features
c) Physiological features | d) Utility of the breed

153. The highest milk yielding breed in India is

a) Jaffarabadi | b) Nili ravi
c) Bhadawari | d) Murrah

154. The following breed of poultry is of Indian origin

a) White leg horn | b) Cornish
c) Aseel | d) Rhode Island red

155. The following is the most prolific goat bred of India

a) Jamanapari | b) Mandya
c) Bengal | d) Chegu

156. In tandem method of selection, the gain per year is maximum, when the numbers of traits, selected are

a) More and negatively correlated
b) More and positively correlated
c) Less and positively correlated
d) Less and negatively correlated

157. The main disadvantage of progeny testing is that

a) It gives little genetic gain
b) The accuracy of the evaluation is not optimum
c) It takes too much time to prove few sires
d) None of the above

158. The genetic progress per generation do not depend on

a) Selection intensity
b) Generation interval
c) Heritability
d) Selection Response

159. The MPPA concept was given by

a) Wright
b) Lush
c) Fisher
d) Pearson

160. The covariance of half-sibs contains

a) ½ VA+1/4 VI+ ....
b) ¼ VA +1/4 DI
c) ¼ VA +1/16 VI+....
d) None of the

161. Close heard is a heard where

a) No female transferred from outside
b) No male transferred to outside
c) Male selected & used within the same herd
d) None of the above

162. Two individuals having same inbreeding coefficient will be

a) Homozygous at the same loci
b) Homozygous at different loci
c) Heterozygous at majority of loci
d) Non of the above

163. Coefficient of inbreeding can be estimated by

a) Path method
b) Tabular method
c) Co ancestry method
d) All the above methods

164. Mercury wool in sheep is characterized by

a) Wool of mercury color
b) Wool with black spots
c) Wool with small balls like appearance
d) None of the above

165. Inbreeding accounts for the homozygosity

a) Alike in descent
b) Alike in state
c) Total Homozygous loci
d) None of the three

166. In criss crossing system of mating we can use

a) Three breeds
b) More than three breeds
c) Two breeds only
d) Only one breed

167. Inbreeding coefficient of an individual produced by mating full sibs is

a) 0.025
b) 0.25
c) 0.50
d) 0.0650

168. In ONBS the replacement female of nucleus are generated from.

a) Nucleus only
b) Cooperating herds only
c) Both1 & 2
d) None of the above

169. If inbreeding coefficient FX of an individual X is 0.250 then coefficient of Relationship of its parent should be

a) 0.50
b) 0.50
c) 0.065
d) None of the above

170. In phenomenon of Heterosis the cross breds

a) Exceeds mid parent
b) Exceeds average of higher parent
c) Exceeds the average of inferior parent
d) All of them

KEY

1. b. Dairy breed
2. c. Gujarat
3. a. Index selection
4. b. Cattle
5. a. Selection
6. b. V_G/V_P
7. a. NDRI, Karnal
8. c. Family selection
9. b. 4 to 4 1/2 Years
10. a. Sunderasan index
11. a. Variance-covariance chart
12. a. Zebu
13. c. Positive assortative mating
14. d. Robert Bakewell
15. c. 25%
16. c. Days open
17. d. Environment
18. b. Pigs
19. b. Dog
20. a. 4-6 generations
21. d. Jersey and Sahiwal
22. b. Negative assortative mating
23. b. 100%
24. a. Ó dy^2
25. c. Line breeding
26. a. Calving interval
27. d. 0 to 1
28. d. All of the above
29. b. Generation interval
30. a. Heterosis
31. d. 56 days
32. d. All the above
33. c. Non additive gene action
34. a. Low heritable traits
35. c. Both a and b
36. a. Toda
37. c. High
38. b. High
39. c. Individual selection
40. a. V_A/V_P
41. c. Frieswal
42. c. Angus
43. c. Is_P
44. a. Repeatability
45. c. Selection
46. b. Holstein Friesian
47. a. Rann of Kutch
48. b. Dairy search index
49. c. Negative
50. b. Kankrej
51. b. Decrease
52. b. Very small
53. c. Individual is
54. c. Hallikar
55. a. Large White Yorkshire
56. b. Uttar Pradesh state
57. c. Tharparkar
58. b. High
59. b. Non-additive gene action
60. a. No genes from collateral relatives
61. a. Superior to tandem method

62. c. Own phenotype
63. a. Tandem method
64. b. Krishnan index
65. c. Draught breed
66. b. Progeny testing
67. c. 1 to 1/2 years
68. a. Independent culling method
69. c. Negative
70. c. Northern England
71. c. Ongole
72. a. Breeding value
73. a. Merino x Nilagiri
74. a. NDRI
75. c. V_{EP} increases
76. c. Identical twins
77. c. Traits with high h^2
78. c. Black Bengal
79. c. Sahiwal
80. d. Poultry
81. b. 0 to +1
82. d. Animal model
83. c. Both a and b
84. a. Chokla
85. c. Holstein-Friesian
86. b. Low
87. b. Progeny testing
88. c. Brown Swiss and Sahiwal
89. c. –1 to +1
90. b. Low
91. b. Superior genotype with best environment
92. c. Spain
93. b. Gaddi
94. d. Mehsana
95. d. Zero
96. b. Family mean
97. c. Karakul
98. a. American class
99. a. 45-60 days
100. c. Generation interval
101. a. England
102. d. France
103. c. Sib testing
104. a. Contemporaries
105. a. Increased variation in the population
106. c. Own phenotype
107. a. Positive
108. b. Repeatability
109. a. Based on phenotype
110. b. Increases the frequencies of desirable genes
111. a. Genotype and phenotype
112. a. Controlled by many genes and are greatly influenced by the environment
113. c. Angora
114. b. Maharashtra

115. b. High
116. d. All the above
117. d. Both b and c
118. a. Depends on the heritability
119. a. 0.4
120. b. Ongole
121. Toda
122. b. 50%
123. c. Heritability
124. a. +1
125. c. Sire index
126. c. Murrah
127. d. Bargur
128. c. Nilgiri
129. b. Selection differential
130. c. Selection index
131. a. Jersey and Holstein Friesian
132. b. Cross breeding
133. c. Species hybridization
134. b. Heterosis
135. a. Coefficient of inbreeding
136. b. Line breeding
137. d. Catello
138. b. Karnal
139. a. Brown Swiss crossbred of Kerala
140. c. Additive gene action
141. b. 0-1
142. d. All
143. a. Deferential
144. c. Both
145. b. Out breeding
146. a. h2 is high
147. a. High h2
148. c. Like-unlike mating
149. a. Jack X Mare
150. a. Rajouri region of J & K
151. c. Hariana
152. c. Physiological features
153. d. Murrah
154. c. Aseel
155. c. Bengal
156. c. Less and positively correlated
157. c. It takes too much time to prove few sires
158. d. Selection Response
159. c. Fisher
160. d. None of the
161. c. Male selected & used within the same herd
162. d. None of the above
163. d. All the above methods
164. c. Wool with small balls like appearance
165. a. Alike in descent
166. c. Two breeds only
167. d. 0.25
168. c. Both 1 & 2
169. b. 0.50
170. a. Exceeds mid parent

4. Match the Most Appropriate

SET I

A	B
a. Jersey	1. Breed of pig
b. Hereford cattle	2. Breed of rabbit
c. Toda	3. Sheep breed
d. Kangayam	4. Goat breed
e. Sunandhini	5. Synthetic sheep breed
f. Mecheri	6. Buffalo breed of Nilgiris
g. Sandyno	7. Beef breed
h. Tellicherry	8. Synthetic breed of cattle
i. Berkshire	9. Exotic milch breed of cattle
j. White Giant	10. Draught Cattle breed
	11. Synthetic goat breed

SET II

A	B
a. Direct relatives	1. Litter size
b. Vembur	2. Carcass yield
c. Sewall Wright	3. 10-15%
d. Collateral relatives	4. Parent-offspring
e. ONBS	5. Inbreeding coefficient
f. J.L. Lush	6. Sheep breed
g. Reproductive trait	7. Coefficient of relationship
h. CNBS	8. Modern animal breeding
i. Prepotency	9. Cousins
j. Sex limited trait	10. Unidirectional
	11. Milk yield

SET III

A	B
a. Longhorn cattle	1. Sibs
b. First stud book	2. Draught purpose cattle breed
c. Multitrait selection	3. Pedigree selection
d. Avikalin	4. Progeny testing
e. MPPA	5. Independent culling method

f. Collateral relatives	6. Robert Bakewell
g. Indirect selection	7. Genetic correlation
h. BLUP	8. Dual purpose cattle breed
i. Large White Yorkshire	9. Synthetic breed of sheep
j. Hariana	10. Breed of pig
	11. Horses
	12. Repeatability

SET IV

A	B
a. Colling brothers	1. $(V_G + V_{EP}) / V_P$
b. Nilsson-Ehle	2. Longhorn cattle
c. Repeatability	3. MPPA
d. Heritability	4. $h_{X.} h_{Y}.r_A$
e. Co-heritability	5. Indirect selection
f. Genetic correlation	6. Quantitative inheritance
g. Selection of cows	7. Bargur
h. Dairy cattle	8. b_{AP}
i. Dual purpose cattle	9. Jersey
j. Draught cattle	10. Shorthorn cattle
	11. Tharparkar
	12. V_E / V_P

SET V

A	B
a. Gir	1. Crossbreed sheep
b. Buffalo	2. Growth rate
c. Sheep	3. Quantitative trait
d. Total score	4. Milch breed
e. Low heritability	5. Qualitative trait
f. Hissardale	6. Jaffarabadi
g. Economic trait	7. Non-additive gene action
h. Horn shape	8. Bikaneri
i. Carcass yield	9. Meat breed of cattle
j. Brangus	10. Method of selection
	11. Draught breed

SET VI

A	B
a. Murrah	1. Carpet wool breed
b. Merino	2. Gujarat state
c. Heritability	3. Milch breed of cattle
d. Surti	4. -1 to + 1
e. Sannen	5. Prominent Roman nose
f. Jaffarabadi	6. Fine wool breed
g. Deccani	7. 0 to 1
h. Genetic correlation	8. Buffalo with sickle shaped horns
i. Jamnapari	9. Exotic milch breed of goat
j. Sahiwal	10. Rohtak

SET VII

A	B
a. Selection index	1. Intermediate index
b. Response to selection	2. Henderson
c. Red Sindhi	3. Shire horses
d. Sundaresan index	4. Total score
e. Intensity of selection	5. R/S
f. Robert Bakewell	6. h2. S
g. BLUP	7. S/sp
h. Equi-parent index	8. Draught breed
i. Hallikar	9. Dairy search index
j. Realized heritability	10. Dairy breed

SET VIII

A	B
a. Sex limited trait	1. 1951
b. First livestock census in British India	2. 1971
c. First livestock census in India after independence	3. One trait at a time
d. First stud book for Throughbred horse in	4. Own phenotype
e. First association for milk recording at	5. Austria
f. Tandem method	6. Denmark

g. Individual selection	7. 1822
h. First trap nesting of laying hens at	8. Several traits
i. Selection index	9. 1919-1920
j. First herd book for shorthorn cattle in	10. Progeny testing

SET IX

A	B
a. Tellicherry	1. Sheep breed in Tamil Nadu
b. Vembur	2. Goat breed of Kerala
c. Jamnapari	3. Sheep breed of Andhra Pradesh
d. Boer	4. Indian breed of poultry
e. White Leghorn	5. Largest goat breed of India
f. Sannen	6. Goat breed in South Africa
g. Azeel	7. Chegu breed of goat
h. Nellore	8. Exotic layer breed of poultry
i. Pashmina	9. Exotic goat breed reared for milk
j. Decanni	10. Exotic milch type cattle
	11. Sheep breed of Maharashtra

SET X

A	B
a. Repeatability	1. J.L.Lush
b. MPPA	2. Dairy search index
c. Heritability of milk yield	3. Goat breed of Tamil Nadu
d. Sire index	4. Intra class correlation
e. Indian dairy breed	5. Sheep breed in Tamil Nadu
f. Kannai Adu	6. 0.2 to 0.3
g. Hereford cattle	7. Sahiwal
h. Mehsana	8. Large White Yorkshire
i. Ramnad White	9. Beef cattle
j. Exotic swine breed	10. Buffalo breed
	11. Robert Bakewell

SET XI

A	B
a. Osborne index	1. Egg size and egg production
b. J.L.Lush	2. High heritability

c. George Coates
d. Krishnan index
e. Mass selection
f. Reproductive traits
g. Negative correlation
h. Robert Bakewell
i. Positive correlation
j. Colling brothers

3. Sire evaluation
4. Milk yield and fat yield
5. Low heritability
6. Selection of poultry
7. Shorthorn cattle
8. Father of modern animal breeding
9. Longhorn cattle
10. First herd book for Shorthorn cattle

SET XII

A

a. Angora goat
b. Plymouth Rock
c. Cornish
d. Law of filial regression
e. Swine
f. Karakul
g, Response to selection
h. Buffalo
i. Ratio of V_{ES} to V_P
j. Correlated response

B

1. Francis Galton
2. Chicken of American origin
3. Sewall wright
4 i $ó_A$h
5. *Bos indicus*
6. 1 – repeatability
7. Mohair production
8. i $h_X r_A ó_{AY}$
9. Chicken of English class
10. *Sus scrofa*
11. i $h^2 ó_P$
12. Fur type sheep breed
13. *Bubalus bubalis*

SET XIII

A

a. Clutch size
b. Commercial tier
c. Cattalo
d. Inbred line
e. CNBS
f. Karan Fries
g. Multiplier tier
h. ONBS
i. Inbreeding
j. Hissardale

B

1. Swine
2. 37.50%
3. Hereditary defects
4. 30-40%
5. Poultry
6. Species hybrid
7. Farmer herd
8. Sheep
9. Crossbred cattle
10. Buffalo

SET XIV

A		B	
a.	Intensity of Selection	1.	One way gene flow
b.	Gurej	2.	Two way gene flow
c.	ONBS	3.	Cross breeding
d.	Out Breeding	4.	h2S
e.	CNBS	5.	Genetic worth of sire
f.	Response to Selection	6.	Differential reproduction
g.	Sire Evaluation	7.	Preservation and upgradation
h.	Inbreeding	8.	Kashmir
i.	Selection	9.	Linebreding
j.	Conservation	10.	z/p

SET XV

A		B	
1.	GCA	a.	Falconer
2.	Milk production	b.	Collateral relatives
3.	Hissardale	c.	Milch goat
4.	Pleiotropy	d.	Nordskog & Kempthrone
5.	Non-additive gene action	e.	Sex limited trait
6.	Yorkshire	f.	Dominance
7.	Jamunapari	g.	Additive gene action
8.	Restricted selection index	h.	Exotic pig
9.	Realized heritability	i.	Genetic correlation
10.	Half sibs	j.	Cross bred sheep

SET XVI

A		B	
a.	Cattlo	1.	Reciprocal of Mule
b.	Crossing of inbred lines	2.	Cross of cattle & buffalo
c.	Rotational Crossing	3.	Diallel Cross
d.	MOET	4.	Heterosis
e.	Data Standardization	5.	Prepotent
f.	Boss Taurus	6.	ONBS
g.	Hinny	7.	Least squares constants
h.	Inbred Sires	8.	Exotic cattle
i.	Inbreeding coefficient	9.	More than three breeds
j.	Non additive gene action	10.	Tabular method

KEY

SET I

	A		B
a.	Jersey	9.	Exotic milch breed of cattle
b.	Hereford cattle	7.	Beef breed
c.	Toda	6.	Buffalo breed of Nilgiris
d.	Kangayam	10.	Draught Cattle breed
e.	Sunandhini	8.	Synthetic breed of cattle
f.	Mecheri	3.	Sheep breed
g.	Sandyno	5.	Synthetic sheep breed
h.	Tellicherry	4.	Goat breed
i.	Berkshire	1.	Breed of pig
j.	White Giant	2.	Breed of rabbit

SET II

	A		B
a.	Direct relatives	4.	Parent-offspring
b.	Vembur	6.	Sheep breed
c.	Sewall Wright	7.	Coefficient of relationship
d.	Collateral relatives	9.	Cousins
e.	ONBS	3.	10-15%
f.	J.L. Lush	8.	Modern animal breeding
g.	Reproductive trait	1.	Litter size
h.	CNBS	10.	Unidirectional
i.	Prepotency	5.	Inbreeding coefficient
j.	Sex limited trait	11.	Milk yield

SET III

	A		B
a.	Longhorn cattle	6.	Robert Bakewell
b.	First stud book	11.	Horses
c.	Multitrait selection	5.	Independent culling method
d.	Avikalin	9.	Synthetic breed of sheep
e.	MPPA	12.	Repeatability
f.	Collateral relatives	1.	Sibs
g.	Indirect selection	7.	Genetic correlation
h.	BLUP	4.	Progeny testing
i.	Large White Yorkshire	10.	Breed of pig
j.	Hariana	8.	Dual purpose cattle breed

SET IV

A	B
a. Colling brothers	10. Shorthorn cattle
b. Nilsson-Ehle	6. Quantitative inheritance
c. Repeatability	1. $(V_G + V_{EP}) / V_P$
d. Heritability	8. b_{AP}
e. Co-heritability	4. $h_X.h_Y.r_A$
f. Genetic correlation	5. Indirect selection
g. Selection of cows	3. MPPA
h. Dairy cattle	9. Jersey
i. Dual purpose cattle	11. Tharparkar
j. Draught cattle	7. Bargur

SET V

A	B
a. Gir	4. Milch breed
b. Buffalo	6. Jaffarabadi
c. Sheep	8. Bikaneri
d. Total score	10. Method of selection
e. Low heritability	7. Non-additive gene action
f. Hissardale	1. Crossbreed sheep
g. Economic trait	3. Quantitative trait
h. Horn shape	5. Qualitative trait
i. Carcass yield	2. Growth rate
j. Brangus	9. Meat breed of cattle

SET VI

A	B
a. Murrah	10. Rohtak
b. Merino	6. Fine wool breed
c. Heritability	7. 0 to 1
d. Surti	8. Buffalo with sickle shaped horns
e. Sannen	9. Exotic milch breed of goat
f. Jaffarabadi	2. Gujarat state
g. Deccani	1. Carpet wool breed
h. Genetic correlation	4. -1 to + 1
i. Jamnapari	5. Prominent Roman nose
j. Sahiwal	3. Milch breed of cattle

SET VII

A	B
a. Selection index	4. Total score
b. Response to selection	6. $h^2.S$
c. Red Sindhi	10. Dairy breed
d. Sundaresan index	9. Dairy search index
e. Intensity of selection	7. S/s_p
f. Robert Bakewell	3. Shire horses
g. BLUP	2. Henderson
h. Equi-parent index	1. Intermediate index
i. Hallikar	8. Draught breed
j. Realized heritability	5. R/S

SET VIII

A	B
a. Sex limited trait	10. Progeny testing
b. First livestock census in British India	9. 1919–1920
c. First livestock census in India after independence	1. 1951
e. First stud book for Throughbred horse in	2. 1971
e. First association for milk recording at	6. Denmark
f. Tandem method	3. One trait at a time
g. Individual selection	4. Own phenotype
h. First trap nesting of laying hens at	5. Austria
i. Selection index	8. Several traits
j. First herd book for shorthorn cattle in	7. 1822

SET IX

A	B
a. Tellicherry	2. Goat breed of Kerala
b. Vembur	1. Sheep breed in Tamil Nadu
c. Jamnapari	5. Largest goat breed of India
d. Boer	6. Goat breed in South Africa
e. White Leghorn	8. Exotic layer breed of poultry

f. Sannen	9. Exotic goat breed reared for milk
g. Azeel	4. Indian breed of poultry
h. Nellore	3. Sheep breed of Andhra Pradesh
i. Pashmina	7. Chegu breed of goat
j. Decanni	11. Sheep breed of Maharashtra

SET X

A	B
b. Repeatability	4. Intra class correlation
b. MPPA	1. J.L.Lush
c. Heritability of milk yield	6. 0.2 to 0.3
d. Sire index	2. Dairy search index
e. Indian dairy breed	7. Gir
f. Kannai Adu	3. Goat breed of Tamil Nadu
g. Hereford cattle	9. Beef cattle
h. Mehsana	10. Buffalo breed
i. Ramnad White	5. Sheep breed in Tamil Nadu
j. Exotic swine breed	8. Large White Yorkshire

SET XI

A	B
a. Osborne index	6. Selection of poultry
b. J.L.Lush	8. Father of modern animal breeding
c. George Coates	10. First herd book for Shorthorn cattle
d. Krishnan index	3. Sire evaluation
e. Mass selection	2. High heritability
f. Reproductive traits	5. Low heritability
g. Negative correlation	1. Egg size and egg production
h. Robert Bakewell	9. Longhorn cattle
i. Positive correlation	4. Milk yield and fat yield
j. Colling brothers	7. Shorthorn cattle

SET XII

A	B
a. Angora goat	7. Mohair production
b. Plymouth Rock	2. Chicken of American origin
c. Cornish	9. Chicken of English class

d. Law of filial regression	1. Francis Galton
e. Swine	10. Sus scrofa
f. Karakul	12. Fur type sheep breed
g, Response to selection	11. $i\ h^2 ó_P$
h. Buffalo	13. *Bubalus bubalis*
i. Ratio of V_{ES} to V_P	6. 1 - repeatability
j. Correlated response	8. $i\ h_X r_A ó_{AY}$

SET XIII

A	B
a. Clutch size	5. Poultry
b. Commercial tier	7. Farmer herd
c. Cattalo	6. Species hybrid
d. Inbred line	2. 37.50%
e. CNBS	1. Swine
f. Karan Fries	9. Crossbred cattle
g. Multiplier tier	4. 30-40%
h. ONBS	10. Buffalo
I. Inbreeding	3. Hereditary defects
j. Hissardale	8. Sheep

SET XIV

A	B
a. Intensity of Selection	10. z/p
b. Gurej	8. Kashmir
c. ONBS	2. Two way gene flow
d. Out Breeding	3. Cross breeding
e. CNBS	1. One way gene flow
f. Response to Selection	4. h2S
g. Sire Evaluation	5. Genetic worth of sire
h. Inbreeding	9. Linebreding
i. Selection	6. Differential reproduction
j. Conservation	7. Preservation and upgradation

SET XV

A	B
1. GCA	g. Additive gene action
2. Milk production	e. Sex limited trait

3.	Hissardale	j.	Cross bred sheep
4.	Pleiotropy	i.	Genetic correlation
5.	Non-additive gene action	f.	Dominance
6.	Yorkshire	h.	Exotic pig
7.	Jamunapari	c.	Milch goat
8.	Restricted selection index	d.	Nordskog & Kempthrone
9.	Realized heritability	a.	Falconer
10.	Half sibs	b.	Collateral relatives

SET XVI

	A		B
a.	Cattlo	2.	Cross of cattle & buffalo
b.	Crossing of inbred lines	3.	Diallel Cross
c.	Rotational Crossing	9.	More than three breeds
d.	MOET	6.	ONBS
e.	Data Standardization	7.	Least squares constants
f.	Boss Taurus	8.	Exotic cattle
g.	Hinny	1.	Reciprocal of Mule
h.	Inbred Sires	5.	Prepotent
i.	Inbreeding coefficient	10.	Tabular method
j.	Non additive gene action	4.	Heterosis

5. Name the Following

1. The class in which the Rhode Island Red breed of poultry belongs.
2. The selection method in which standards are fixed for each trait.
3. The indigenous breed of fowl noted for its fighting quality.
4. The record of an individual's ancestors.
5. The raw material for selection.
6. The product of selection differential and heritability.
7. The crossing in which breeds or strains are mated in all possible combinations.
8. The value of an individual judged by mean value of its parents.
9. Gene action responsible for general combining ability.
10. The measure of variation in a trait in a population.

11. The breed of buffalo evolved by crossing Murrah and Surti.
12. An example to indicate the G X E interaction.
13. The method of selection in which economic weights is considered.
14. Regression of breeding value on phenotypic value.
15. The fiber obtained from Angora goats.
16. The standardized selection differential.
17. Home tract / State of the following breeds of livestock and poultry. Sahiwal, Tharparkar, Gir, Ongole, Khillari, Murrah, Surti buffalo, Toda, Nali, Mandya, Beetal, Barbari, Sirohi, Osmanabadi, Plymouth Rock, New Hampshire, Cornish, Azeel, Kadaknath.
18. Breeds used for evolving the following new breeds.
19. Jamaica Hope, Australian milking zebu, Karan Fries, Karan Swiss, Sunandhini, Avikalin, Sandyno, Hissardale, Avivastra.
20. Two new breeds of sheep developed in CSWRI, Avikanagar.

6. Expand the Following

1. AICRP
2. AMUL
3. AnGR
4. BLUP
5. CIRG
6. CSWRI
7. DAD-IS
8. DHIA
9. ETT
10. FAO
11. FPT
12. GCA
13. ICDP
14. IVF
15. IVM
16. IVRI
17. KVS
18. MAS
19. MOET
20. NBAGR
21. NDDB
22. NDRI
23. NPCBB
24. NRC
25. PBV
26. PDC
27. CIRC
28. QTL
29. RAPD
30. RFLP
31. SCA

7. Define the Following

1. Dominance
2. Breed
3. Inbreeding coefficient
4. Lactation length
5. Random mating or Panmixia
6. Top crossing
7. Selective breeding
8. Diallel crossing
9. Animal breeding
10. Synthetic or composite breed
11. Animal breeding
12. Brangus
13. Breed
14. Breeding value
15. Bull is half the herd
16. Correlated response
17. Common environmental effects / c-effects
18. Cross-covariance
19. Culling
20. Diallele crossing
21. Estimated breeding value (EBV)
22. Family selection
23. General combining ability
24. Generation interval
25. Genetic antagonism
26. Genetic trend
27. Genetic load
28. Genetic gain

29. Heritability
30. Heterosis
31. Inbred line
32. Mass selection
33. Natural selection
34. Pedigree
35. Phenotype
36. Prepotency
37. Realized heritability
38. Repeatability
39. Response to selection
40. Selection differential
41. Selection index
42. Selection limit
43. Sire index
44. Specific combining ability
45. Standardized selection differential
46. Strain
47. Stud book
48. Truncation selection
49. Trait ratio
50. Dry period

8. Differentiate the Following

1. Back cross and test cross
2. Basis of selection and Methods of selection
3. Close inbreeding and line breeding
4. CNBS and ONBS
5. Conservation and preservation

6. Crossbreeding and grading up
7. Direct and collateral relatives
8. Family selection and sib selection
9. General and specific combining ability
10. Generation interval and calving interval
11. Genetic and operational complications of selection
12. Genus and species
13. Half sib and full sib
14. Herdmate and contemporaries
15. Heritability and repeatability
16. Heritability in broad and narrow sense
17. Heterosis and complementarity
18. Heterosis and inbreeding depression
19. Inbreeding and outbreeding
20. Inbreeding coefficient and relationship coefficient
21. Incrossing and In cross breeding
22. Independent culling level and index selection
23. *In-situ* and *ex-situ* conservation
24. *In-vivo* and *In-vitro* methods of conservation
25. Line and strain
26. Line breeding and line crossing
27. Mohair and Pashmina
28. Multistage and multisource selection index
29. Natural and artificial selection
30. Out breeding and out crossing
31. Pedigree selection and progeny testing
32. Phenotypic correlation and genetic correlation
33. Positive and negative assortative mating
34. Random mating and non-random mating

35. Recurrent and reciprocal recurrent selection
36. Selection and culling
37. Selection differential and selection intensity
38. Selection response and selection plateau
39. Strain and Inbred line
40. Tandem and total score method

9. Write Short Notes on the Following

1. Principles of Robert Bakewell
2. MPPA
3. Restricted selection index
4. Dairy breeds of Indian cattle
5. Galton's law of filial regression
6. Cattle and buffalo breeding policy of Tamil Nadu state
7. What is conservation? Describe different methods of conservation.
8. Nucleus breeding schemes
9. Genetic basis of Heterosis or hybrid vigour
10. Breed formation
11. Record keeping
12. Breeding strategies for genetic improvement of goats
13. Synthetic breeds of dairy cattle developed in India
14. Types of conservation of animal genetic resources
15. Cattle and buffalo breeding policy of India
16. Standardization of lactation records
17. Reasons for outbreeding
18. Categories of uniparous domestic populations according to vulnerability
19. Synthetic breed
20. Specific and rotational crossing
21. Development of inbred lines

22. Reasons for conservation
23. Accuracy of selection in progeny testing
24. Advantages of family selection
25. Any three draught breeds of Indian cattle
26. Any two breeds of buffalo
27. Asymmetry of response
28. Breed characteristics of Sahiwal, Tharparkar / Gir, Kangayam
29. BLUP
30. Boer goat
31. Casual and observational components of phenotypic variance
32. Classification of breeds of chicken based on utility with example
33. Classification of breeds of ducks based on utility with example
34. Combined selection
35. Corrected daughter average index
36. Correlated response
37. Dairy breeds of Indian cattle
38. Dairy search index
39. Diallele crossing
40. Describe the uses and limitations of progeny testing
41. Economic traits of meat type sheep
42. Equi-parent index
43. Estimation of heritability by sib analysis
44. Exotic breeds of sheep/goats/pigs used in India with its breed characteristics
45. Factors affecting selection differential
46. Factors affecting selection progress/response to selection
47. Family selection
48. Galton's law of filial regression
49. Genetic correlation and its application in animal breeding

50. Genetic gain
51. Genotype X Environment interaction
52. Hairy meat breeds of sheep in India
53. Herd book
54. Herd-mate comparison
55. Heritability
56. How repeatability is useful in selection of cows for high milk production
57. Importance of phenotypic variation
58. Independent culling method of selection
59. Indirect selection
60. Individual selection
61. Intensity of selection
62. Indian breeds of chicken
63. Jamaica Hope cattle
64. Krishnan's index
65. Mecheri sheep
66. MPPA
67. Murrah, Surti and Nili-Ravi breeds of buffalo
68. Mysore breeds of cattle
69. Osborne index
70. Pedigree selection and its limitations
71. Pedigree sheets
72. Principles of Robert Bakewell
73. Precision in the estimation of heritability
74. Probable breeding value
75. Procedure for evolving a new breed of dairy cattle
76. Progeny testing
77. Realized heritability
78. Types of heterosis

79. Reciprocal recurrent selection
80. Recurrent selection
81. Red Sindhi
82. Species hybridization
83. Requirements for construction of selection index
84. Response to selection/genetic gain
85. Selection index
86. Selection limit/selection plateau
87. Selection differential
88. Sib selection
89. Sire index
90. Sheep breeds of Tamil Nadu
91. Superior carpet wool breeds of sheep in India
92. Synthetic/new breeds of cattle in India
93. Synthetic/new breeds of sheep in India
94. Tandem method of selection
95. Trait ratio
96. Uses of heritability estimates
97. Uses of repeatability estimates
98. Exotic breeds of cattle used in India for breeding
99. Mysore breeds of cattle
100. Classification of goat breeds based on region
101. Classification of poultry breeds according to the region
102. Indigenous breeds of poultry

10. Write Essay on the Following

1. Define heritability. Explain different methods of estimation of heritability with the principle involved and write the practical uses of heritability in animal breeding programme.
2. a) Describe in details about the different methods of multi-trait selection in farm animals with merits and demerits of each.

   b) What are the different measures of selection response?
3. Define general and specific combining ability. Give various breeding plans for utilizing general and specific combining ability for improving egg production in chicken.
4. What is inbreeding? Explain the different types of inbreeding and its genetic and phenotypic effects
5. Define economic trait. Describe various economic traits in dairy cattle
6. Define crossbreeding. Explain in brief the different methods of crossbreeding. Write the advantages and disadvantages of crossbreeding.
7. Define GCA and SCA. Describe in detail the method of reciprocal recurrent selection in poultry production
8. Write in detail the various economic traits in buffalo
9. What are the genetic parameters estimated for different traits in farm animals? Explain the applications of each in animal breeding programme.
10. Define heritability. Explain different methods of estimation of heritability with the principle involved and write the practical uses heritability in animal breeding programme.
11. a) What is repeatability? How is it calculated?

    b) What are the uses of repeatability in animal breeding programmes?.
12. Why correlated characters are important in genetic studies? Write brief essay on genetic, environmental and phenotypic correlations.
13. Define genetic correlation. Establish the relationship among phenotypic, genetic and environmental correlations. Describe the estimation of genetic correlation and its uses. Describe the difference between positive and negative genetic correlation with suitable examples.
14. a) Define selection. Describe different methods of multi trait selection in animal breeding. Indicate the merits and demerits of each method.

    b) Write in short about the most efficient method of multi trait selection

15. a) Describe in details about the different methods of multi-trait selection in farm animals with merits and demerits of each.

    b) What are the different measures of selection response?

16. Explain in detail the best method of selection listing out the different methods.

17. Explain the method of selection, which gives due weightage to the traits considered and mention the other methods over which it is superior.

18. What are the different aids available for selection? Discuss the principles and procedure for progeny testing in cattle and precautions to be taken while estimating the breeding values of sires.

19. Enumerate different aids to selection? Discuss combined selection with an example.

20. What are the different aids to selection? Describe selection on the basis of progeny testing with its advantages and limitations.

21. What are the different aids to selection? Describe selection where the records of individual's ancestors are considered.

22. What are the different aids to selection? Indicate the merits and demerits of each method.

23. What is response to selection? Discuss the factors affecting response per unit of time (year) and selection limit.

24. Describe Recurrent Selection and Reciprocal Recurrent Selection.

25. Define general and specific combining ability. Give various breeding plans for utilizing general and specific combining ability for improving egg production in chicken.

26. Define Sire Index. List out the methods to estimate it and discuss on recent and better method of sire evaluation. Write in detail on contemporary comparison.

27. What is Sire Index? Enumerate the different methods and explain in detail the method developed by Henderson

28. Write an essay on genotype X environment interaction.

29. a) Define breed and describe the breed characteristics of Zebu cattle.

    b) Classify the breeds of cattle in India based on utility and describe the characteristics of each one dairy, draught and dual-purpose breed.

30. Write the origin, breed characteristics including traits of economic importance of

    a) two exotic cattle breeds exclusively used for crossbreeding in India.

    b) two Indian buffalo breeds.

31. List the important milch breeds of cattle in India and describe their distribution, breed characteristics in detail.

32. Classify the breeds of sheep and goats in India based on their utility and describe any five important meat breeds of sheep and goats each indicating their home tract, breed characteristics and distinguishing features.

33. Classify the breeds of fowls in the world and give two examples in each. Discuss the breed characteristics of White Leghorn.

34. a) What are the reasons for new breed formation

    b) Give steps for evolving a new breed of dairy cattle suitable for low lands of South India.

35. List the traits of economic importance in dairy cattle/meat type sheep and explain how each of it can be improved.

❑❑❑